The Two Faces of Nanomaterials

The Two Faces of Nanomaterials: Toxicity and Bioactivity

Special Issue Editors

Dong-Wook Han
Timur Sh. Atabaev

MDPI • Basel • Beijing • Wuhan • Barcelona • Belgrade • Manchester • Tokyo • Cluj • Tianjin

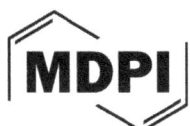

Special Issue Editors

Dong-Wook Han
Pusan National University (PNU)
Korea

Timur Sh. Atabaev
Nazarbayev University
Kazakhstan

Editorial Office
MDPI
St. Alban-Anlage 66
4052 Basel, Switzerland

This is a reprint of articles from the Special Issue published online in the open access journal *Nanomaterials* (ISSN 2079-4991) (available at: https://www.mdpi.com/journal/nanomaterials/special_issues/toxi_biotoxicity).

For citation purposes, cite each article independently as indicated on the article page online and as indicated below:

LastName, A.A.; LastName, B.B.; LastName, C.C. Article Title. *Journal Name* **Year**, *Article Number*, Page Range.

ISBN 978-3-03928-983-7 (Hbk)
ISBN 978-3-03928-984-4 (PDF)

Cover image courtesy of Bong Joo Park.

© 2020 by the authors. Articles in this book are Open Access and distributed under the Creative Commons Attribution (CC BY) license, which allows users to download, copy and build upon published articles, as long as the author and publisher are properly credited, which ensures maximum dissemination and a wider impact of our publications.

The book as a whole is distributed by MDPI under the terms and conditions of the Creative Commons license CC BY-NC-ND.

Contents

About the Special Issue Editors vii

Preface to "The Two Faces of Nanomaterials: Toxicity and Bioactivity" ix

Iruthayapandi Selestin Raja, Su-Jin Song, Moon Sung Kang, Yu Bin Lee, Bongju Kim, Suck Won Hong, Seung Jo Jeong, Jae-Chang Lee and Dong-Wook Han
Toxicity of Zero- and One-Dimensional Carbon Nanomaterials
Reprinted from: *Nanomaterials* **2019**, *9*, 1214, doi:10.3390/nano9091214 1

Qian Li, Chun Huang, Liwei Liu, Rui Hu and Junle Qu
Effect of Surface Coating of Gold Nanoparticles on Cytotoxicity and Cell Cycle Progression
Reprinted from: *Nanomaterials* **2018**, *8*, 1063, doi:10.3390/nano8121063 25

Su-Jin Song, Yong Cheol Shin, Hyun Uk Lee, Bongju Kim, Dong-Wook Han and Dohyung Lim
Dose- and Time-Dependent Cytotoxicity of Layered Black Phosphorus in Fibroblastic Cells
Reprinted from: *Nanomaterials* **2018**, *8*, 408, doi:10.3390/nano8060408 39

Eloisa Ferrone, Rodolfo Araneo, Andrea Notargiacomo, Marialilia Pea and Antonio Rinaldi
ZnO Nanostructures and Electrospun ZnO–Polymeric Hybrid Nanomaterials in Biomedical, Health, and Sustainability Applications
Reprinted from: *Nanomaterials* **2019**, *9*, 1449, doi:10.3390/nano9101449 49

Elsie Zurob, Geraldine Dennett, Dana Gentil, Francisco Montero-Silva, Ulrike Gerber, Pamela Naulín, Andrea Gómez, Raúl Fuentes, Sheila Lascano, Thiago Henrique Rodrigues da Cunha, Cristian Ramírez, Ricardo Henríquez, Valeria del Campo, Nelson Barrera, Marcela Wilkens and Carolina Parra
Inhibition of Wild *Enterobacter cloacae* Biofilm Formation by Nanostructured Graphene- and Hexagonal Boron Nitride-Coated Surfaces
Reprinted from: *Nanomaterials* **2019**, *9*, 49, doi:10.3390/nano9010049 83

Kyong-Hoon Choi, Ki Chang Nam, Guangsup Cho, Jin-Seung Jung and Bong Joo Park
Enhanced Photodynamic Anticancer Activities of Multifunctional Magnetic Nanoparticles (Fe_3O_4) Conjugated with Chlorin e6 and Folic Acid in Prostate and Breast Cancer Cells
Reprinted from: *Nanomaterials* **2018**, *8*, 722, doi:10.3390/nano8090722 101

Natalja Fjodorova, Marjana Novič, Katja Venko and Bakhtiyor Rasulev
A Comprehensive Cheminformatics Analysis of Structural Features Affecting the Binding Activity of Fullerene Derivatives
Reprinted from: *Nanomaterials* **2020**, *10*, 90, doi:10.3390/nano10010090 111

About the Special Issue Editors

Dong-Wook Han (Prof.) obtained his B.S. in the Department of Biochemistry at Yonsei University, Seoul, in 1998. He completed his M.S. and Ph.D. degrees in the graduate program of biomedical engineering from Yonsei University in 2000 and 2004, respectively. With two and a half years of experience as a postdoctoral fellow (under the supervision of Prof. Suong-Hyu Hyon) at the Institute for Frontier Medical Sciences, Kyoto University, Japan, Dr. Han returned to Korea. In 2008, he joined the faculty of Pusan National University (PNU) where he began his academic career as an assistant professor and is currently a full professor and chair in the Department of Optics and Mechatronics Engineering at PNU. Dr. Han is serving as a board member of several biomedical societies and an editorial board member of many scientific journals including BioMed Research International, Nanomaterials, World Journal of Stem Cells, Journal of Nanotheranostics, Biomaterials Research, etc. Since 2008, he has authored or co-authored over 120 scientific publications, possesses over 10 international and national patents, and jointly authored several book chapters. His research interest concerns BT–NT convergence, especially tissue engineering and regenerative/translational medicine using smart nanobiomaterials; development of artificial tissues/organs, medical devices, and organs-on-chips; 3D bioprinting; cell imaging; and evaluation of biocompatibility and nanotoxicity.

Timur Sh. Atabaev (Assistant Prof.) received his Ph.D. degree (nanoscience and nanotechnology, under the supervision of Profs. Yoon-Hwae Hwang and Hyung Kook Kim) at Pusan National University (South Korea) in 2012. From 2012 to 2017, he worked as a postdoctoral fellow and research professor both at Pusan National University and Seoul National University. Since 2017, he has been an Assistant Professor in Chemistry at Nazarbayev University, Kazakhstan. His areas of specialization include multifunctional materials and advanced nanostructures for biomedical, optical, energy, sensing, and photocatalytic applications. He has delivered several invited talks and served as a committee member for numerous international meetings. He is a member of the American Chemical Society and Royal Society of Chemistry. He was a recipient of the Young Researcher of the Year Scopus 2018 award.

Preface to "The Two Faces of Nanomaterials: Toxicity and Bioactivity"

Since the early 2000s, a growing number of nanomaterials (NMs) have received attention due to the advances in nanomedicine, including the use of various nanoparticles for therapeutic and diagnostic purposes. NMs have different properties compared with larger materials, and these properties can be used in a wide spectrum of biomedical areas, such as theragnosis, drug delivery, imaging, sensing, and tissue engineering. In this context, the safety (or toxicity) profile of NMs and their impact on health must be evaluated to attain their biocompatibility and desired activity for their development. However, certain controversies remain. Despite certain inconsistencies in several detailed experimental results from numerous reports, some in vitro and in vivo studies clearly showed no particular risks posed by NMs, whereas others have indicated that NMs might become health hazards.

In this book, two review papers and five original research works focus on a better understanding the correlation of the biological effects of NMs with their intrinsic physicochemical and thermomechanical properties. This book provides novel scientific findings on the bioactivity of NMs and some perspectives on potential risks to their future development in biomedical science and engineering as well as potential applications to various clinical fields.

Dong-Wook Han, Timur Sh. Atabaev
Special Issue Editors

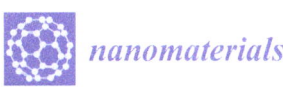

Review

Toxicity of Zero- and One-Dimensional Carbon Nanomaterials

Iruthayapandi Selestin Raja [1,†], Su-Jin Song [2,†], Moon Sung Kang [2], Yu Bin Lee [2], Bongju Kim [3], Suck Won Hong [2], Seung Jo Jeong [4], Jae-Chang Lee [5,*] and Dong-Wook Han [2,*]

1. Monocrystalline Bank Research Institute, Pusan National University, Busan 46241, Korea
2. Department of Cogno-Mechatronics Engineering, College of Nanoscience & Nanotechnology, Pusan National University, Busan 46241, Korea
3. Dental Life Science Research Institute & Clinical Translational Research Center for Dental Science, Seoul National University Dental Hospital, Seoul 03080, Korea
4. GS Medical Co., Ltd., Cheongju-si, Chungcheongbuk-do 28161, Korea
5. Bio-Based Chemistry Research Center, Korea Research Institute of Chemical Technology, Ulsan 44429, Korea
* Correspondence: jclee@krict.re.kr (J.-C.L.); nanohan@pusan.ac.kr (D.-W.H.)
† These authors contributed equally to this work.

Received: 5 August 2019; Accepted: 23 August 2019; Published: 28 August 2019

Abstract: The zero (0-D) and one-dimensional (1-D) carbon nanomaterials have gained attention among researchers because they exhibit a larger surface area to volume ratio, and a smaller size. Furthermore, carbon is ubiquitously present in all living organisms. However, toxicity is a major concern while utilizing carbon nanomaterials for biomedical applications such as drug delivery, biosensing, and tissue regeneration. In the present review, we have summarized some of the recent findings of cellular and animal level toxicity studies of 0-D (carbon quantum dot, graphene quantum dot, nanodiamond, and carbon black) and 1-D (single-walled and multi-walled carbon nanotubes) carbon nanomaterials. The in vitro toxicity of carbon nanomaterials was exemplified in normal and cancer cell lines including fibroblasts, osteoblasts, macrophages, epithelial and endothelial cells of different sources. Similarly, the in vivo studies were illustrated in several animal species such as rats, mice, zebrafish, planktons and, guinea pigs, at various concentrations, route of administrations and exposure of nanoparticles. In addition, we have described the unique properties and commercial usage, as well as the similarities and differences among the nanoparticles. The aim of the current review is not only to signify the importance of studying the toxicity of 0-D and 1-D carbon nanomaterials, but also to emphasize the perspectives, future challenges and possible directions in the field.

Keywords: carbon nanomaterials; unique properties; biomedical applications; in vitro toxicity; in vivo toxicity

1. Introduction

Nanotechnology has been a rapidly developing field, producing many nanomaterials with alterations in different physical and physicochemical properties such as size, shape, crystalline nature, and interaction with biological systems [1–3]. These materials have found adaptability in biomedical applications such as nanomedicines, cosmetics, bioelectronics, biosensors, and biochips [4]. However, the fact that possible health risks are associated with the increasing development of nanotechnology cannot be set aside. Nanoparticles may be either organic or inorganic based on the composition of elements. Mostly, inorganic nanomaterials are based on transition metals such as silver, iron, gold, zinc, copper, etc. whereas carbon nanomaterials are mainly composed of the carbon element, which constitutes various spatial arrangements in different nanoscales from zero (0-D) to three dimensions (3-D) [1,5–7]. In the present review, we will discuss the toxicity of 0-D carbon nanostructures (carbon black, nanodiamond, carbon nanodots and fullerene) and 1-D nanomaterials (single and multi-walled carbon nanotubes) from the research that has been conducted over the past two decades. The structure of carbon nanomaterials is shown in Figure 1.

Carbon dots are carbon-based nanomaterials with unique properties such as chemical inertness, optical stability, and wavelength-dependent photoluminescence [8]. Carbon quantum dots (CQDs) are typically quasi-spherical nanoparticles with a diameter less than 10 nm and composed of carbon, oxygen, hydrogen, nitrogen, and other elements. Because of their hydrophilic nature and cell permeation, CQDs have replaced traditional metal-based quantum dots in many applications, including photovoltaics, photocatalysis, and drug targeting [9]. The oxidized CQDs may contain 5–50% oxygen depending on synthetic procedures. Carbon quantum dots typically present two optical absorption bands in the UV-vis spectrum, which are attributed to π–π^* and n–π^* transitions in C=C and C=O bonds, respectively [10]. When the carbon nanodots are represented as a π-conjugated single sheet, with a size of 2–10 nm, they are called graphene quantum dots [11]. It has been reported that graphene quantum dots (GQDs) exhibit magnetic, electronic, and optical properties [12].

Nanodiamonds (NDs) are carbon-based crystalline nanoparticles inheriting diamond structure at the nanoscale with excellent properties such as optical transparency, hardness and chemical inertness [13]. The sp^3 tetrahedral structure of the nanodiamond presents Raman signal at 1332 cm^{-1} and is capable of fluorescing due to point defects. However, the non-fluorescing nanodiamond displays a strong coherent anti-Stokes Raman scattering effect [14]. The quantitative analysis of cellular uptake of NDs is promising for the applications of bio labeling and bio imaging. The oxidized form of the nanodiamond has been reported to damage DNA in embryonic stem cells [15].

Carbon black nanoparticles (CBNPs) are the zero-dimensional carbon-based nanomaterials, which are produced in large quantities in different ways, such as partial combustion and thermal decomposition of hydrocarbons either in liquid or gaseous state [16]. The poor water-soluble carbon black poses a threat to health when exposed to the lungs through inhalation. The core portion of the insoluble particle yields reactive oxygen species (ROS), which render toxicity to the experimental animals [17]. Recently, the International Agency for Research on Cancer (IARC) listed carbon black nanoparticles as carcinogenic to human beings [16]. In toxicological studies, carbon black nanoparticles (CBNPs), with diameters less than 100 nm, have been reference material for diesel exhaust particles [18]. The aciniform aggregates of carbon black are basically fine powder in the size range of 100–1000 nm in a closed reaction chamber and form larger agglomerates due to van der Waals forces in the final step of the manufacturing process [19]. The term 'carbon black' should not be confused with such words as black carbon and soot, which are the carbonaceous materials emitted from incomplete combustion of fuels, such as waste oil, diesel, gasoline, wood, paper, plastic and rubber [20]. It is important to note that carbon black nanoparticles have certain physicochemical properties in common with another insoluble carbonaceous material, including graphene [16]. CBNPs have been widely used as conductive fillers due to their low aspect ratio, being economically inexpensive, and having good conductivity [21,22].

Among the carbon-based nanomaterials, fullerene (C60) is a generic term for a cluster composed of 60 carbon atoms that appears as a soccer-ball structure. The C60 contains 30 carbon atoms to readily interact with free radicals, and therefore is known as a free radical sponge [23,24]. The versatile applications of C60 include use in superconducting devices, energy device materials and catalysts [25]. The water-soluble polyhydroxylated fullerene, known as fullerenol (C60(OH)n), has been explored for its potential as being an anticancer, anti-HIV and skin rejuvenating cosmetic [25,26]. Fullerenol was reported to protect experimental animals from hepatotoxicity and doxorubicin-induced cardiotoxicity [26,27]. In nature, fullerene is available as its analogues including C70, C80, and C94, because of its tendency to aggregate and form a crystal-like structure with a diameter of 100 nm [23]. The research studies revealed that skin contact and nasal inhalation are the most likely routes of exposure to fullerenes for the workers in industries [25].

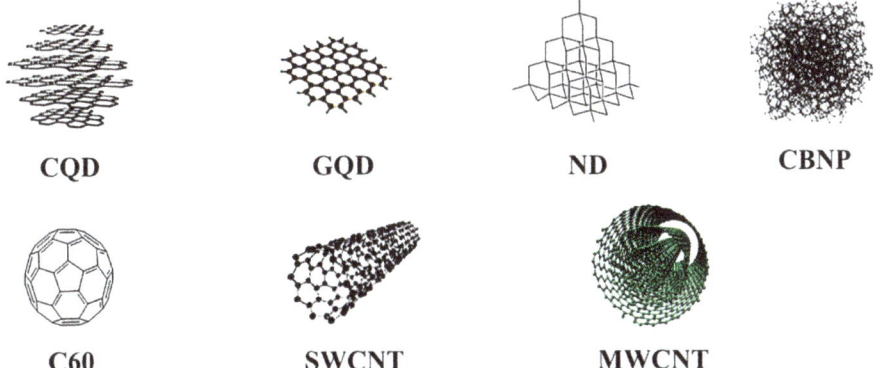

Figure 1. The structure of zero- and one-dimensional carbon nanomaterials have been shown. Carbon quantum dot (CQD) and graphene quantum dot (GQD), reproduced with permission from [11], Copyright Royal Society of Chemistry, 2010; nanodiamond (ND) and fullerene (C60), reproduced with permission from [7], Copyright American Chemical Society, 2013; carbon black nanoparticle (CBNP), reproduced with permission from [28], Copyright Elsevier, 2014; single-walled carbon nanotube (SWCNT) and multi-walled carbon nanotube (MWCNT), reproduced with permission from [29], Copyright Elsevier, 2017.

The unique property of CNT is its high aspect ratio, which promotes its superior properties to the encapsulating matrix polymers and has advantages over traditional reinforcements [30]. The most widely used techniques for the synthesis of carbon nanotubes (CNTs) are laser furnace, chemical vapor deposition, and arc discharge [31]. Their biomedical applications include biosensors, orthopedic prostheses, anticancer therapy, and tissue engineering [32]. The literature reports reveal that maternal exposure of CNTs might develop developmental toxicity such as teratogenicity [33]. The threat of nanotoxicity of CNTs is an increasing trend, as the global production of CNTs reaches several thousand tons per year [32]. Based on morphology, the carbon nanotube is generally classified into the two viz. single-walled and multi-walled carbon nanotubes. When one or several graphene sheets are rolled up to a cylindrical form concentrically, they yield single-walled carbon nanotubes (SWCNTs) and multi-walled carbon nanotubes (MWCNTs), respectively. Meanwhile, MWCNTs differ from SWCNTs in some physicochemical properties, such as the number of layers, the surface area and width [34,35]. The preparation of both CNTs also varies with different experimental conditions. For example, in the electric arc discharge method, SWCNTs are synthesized in the form of soot when a graphite rod comprising a metal catalyst acts as an anode and pure graphite as a cathode. Meanwhile, the production of MWCNTs is achieved strictly in the presence of inert gas such as helium. In the laser vaporization method, generation of SWCNTs mainly depends on the type of metal catalyst and the furnace temperature, whereas the yield of MWCNTs requires a pure graphite target and an optimum temperature of 1200 °C [36]. The nanotubes strongly interact with each other by van der Waals forces and hence exhibit hydrophobicity, which limits their biomedical applications. Hypochlorite, myeloperoxidase, and eosinophils peroxidase have been reported to degrade nanotubes within phagosomes and in the inflammation sites [37]. Researchers have adopted different approaches to modify pristine CNTs to impart hydrophilic behavior. The π-conjugated skeleton of CNT was covalently modified through different chemical reactions such as sidewall halogenation, hydrogenation, plasma activation, cycloaddition, radical, nucleophilic and electrophilic additions. The non-covalent modification occurs by physical attachment of various functional molecules and the endohedral filling takes place at the inner empty cavity of CNT [38].

SWCNTs have been used in a wide range of commercial applications such as earthquake-resistant buildings, dent-resistant car bodies, stain-resistant textiles and transistors [39]. The diameter of

SWCNTs is approximately 1–2 nm and their toxicity is more substantial in comparison to MWCNTs (10–20 nm) and other carbonaceous nanomaterials such as carbon black and fullerene [40]. Despite being an attractive structural material with a high aspect ratio of length to width, carbon nanotubes threaten living organisms with potentially hazardous effects [41]. As far as the drug administration of SWCNTs is concerned, the inhalation route of exposure has more serious effects than the aspiration route in terms of oxidative stress, inflammatory responses, fibrosis and collagen deposition [42]. It has been reported that the agglomerates of SWCNTs caused granulomas in the proximal alveoli, and dispersed SWCNTs instigated interstitial fibrosis in the distal alveoli [43]. Similar to asbestos, MWCNTs have been reported to possess pathogenicity, owing to their larger durability and needle-like shape [32]. They found a wide variety of industrial applications in rechargeable batteries, water filters and sporting goods [44]. It was informed that non-branched MWCNTs had a higher potential to cause mesothelioma than the tangled MWCNTs [45].

2. In Vitro Cellular Toxicity of Zero- and One-Dimensional Carbon Nanomaterials

The in vitro toxicity effects of carbon nanomaterials (0-D and 1-D) have been listed in Table 1. The cytotoxic effect of the polyethylenimine (PEI) coated CQDs based nanohybrid, with a diameter of 6.5 ± 2 nm, was investigated at various concentrations (200, 400, 600 and 800 µg/mL) on kidney epithelial cells derived from the African green monkey. The MTT (3-(4,5-dimethylthiazol-2-yl)-2,5-diphenyltetrazolium bromide) assay revealed that the nanohybrid killed 39% of cells at concentration 600 µg/mL, despite there being no sign of significant toxicity at lower concentrations [46]. The pristine fluorescent carbon quantum dots (~7 nm) were evaluated for its cytotoxicity assessing total ROS, glutathione, and lactate dehydrogenase activity on human bronchial epithelial cells (16 HBE). The data revealed that CQDs preferentially located on the surface of cells and that its exposure induced oxidative stress and decreased cell viability [47]. A comprehensive study was presented to describe the critical role of functionalized nanoparticles in cytotoxicity using mouse embryonic fibroblasts (NIH-3T3). The CQDs synthesized from candle soot were negatively charged. The pristine CQDs were then functionalized with PEG (polyethylene glycol) and PEI to impart neutral and positive charges on the surface of nanoparticles, respectively. The results of in vitro cellular toxicity measurements revealed that the neutral charged CQDs did not induce any abnormalities in the cell cycle, cellular trafficking and cell morphology up to the concentrations of 300 µg/mL. Meanwhile, the negatively charged pristine CQDs arrested the cell cycle at the G2/M phase, enhanced cell proliferation, and caused oxidative stress. Being the most cytotoxic, the positively charged CQDs triggered a significant alteration in the cell cycle at the G0/G1 phase, at a concentration of 100 µg/mL [48].

GQDs have also shown different cellular uptake in MC3T3 osteoblast cell lines derived from mouse calvaria and exhibited low cytotoxicity due to their small size and high oxygen content [49]. The adverse effects of hydroxyl-modified GQDs (OH-GQDs) were studied on human lung carcinoma cell lines H1299 and A549. The OH-GQDs with hydrodynamic diameter of 10.3 ± 1.9 nm, at a concentration 50 µg/mL, decreased cell viability and intracellular ROS generation at a significant level. The cell signaling pathway analysis exposed that hydroxylated GQDs induced G0/G1 arrest, cell senescence, and inhibition of Rb phosphorylation in both types of cells [50]. It was confirmed that GQDs were less cytotoxic to human breast cancer (MCF-7) and human gastric cancer (MGC-803) cells on prolonged incubation. The nanoparticles significantly permeated into both cytoplasm and nucleus of the cells following caveolae-mediated endocytosis, but they did not affect cellular morphology. In addition, the nanoparticles exhibited lower cytotoxicity to MGC-803 cells when compared to MCF-7 cells [51].

Genotoxicity of NDs was analyzed on mouse embryonic stem cells and the results revealed that NDs of 4–5 nm expressed an elevated level of DNA repair proteins such as p53 and MOGG-1. Further, oxidized NDs were described to have more influence on triggering DNA damage than the pristine NDs. However, it was demonstrated that NDs, either in oxidized form or pristine, were not severe in toxicity when compared to MWCNTs [52]. Intracellular ROS, mitochondrial activity, apoptosis, colony formation, and cellular uptake were studied to provide elucidative information about the toxicity of NDs in two different cell lines HaCaT and A549. At concentration of 1.0 mg/mL, inhibition of colony formation and small degree apoptosis were observed in cells. However, it was found that NDs did not have any significant influence on cell viability and ROS production [53]. Treated with RAW 264.7 murine macrophages, the cytotoxicity of NDs were examined in various sizes (6–500 nm) and concentrations (0–200 µg/mL). Cell proliferation and metabolic activity were found reduced in a concentration dependent manner. Flow cytometry analysis revealed that the nanoparticles caused necrosis, leading to significant cytotoxicity, irrespective of particle size [54]. In vitro toxicity measurements were carried out in human blood cells and the reports exposed that NDs could change the kinetics of active oxygen production, cause erythrocyte hemolysis and destruct white cells [55].

The in vitro genotoxic and mutagenic potential of NDs were investigated in human lymphocytes and the nanoparticles were reported to inhibit cell proliferation-inducing apoptotic cell death above 50 µg/mL. The cellular oxidative stress generated by the nanoparticles was found to be dose-dependent. Significant changes in chromatin stability followed by DNA oxidative damage were established, even at a concentration of 1 µg/mL. NDs had the potential to stimulate micronuclei augmenting centromeric signals at 10 µg/mL [56]. The viability of human umbilical vein endothelial cells (HUVEC-ST) was investigated following the treatment of NDs, which was synthesized by the detonation method. The results of the MTT assay revealed that NDs showed a concentration-dependent cytotoxicity and ROS production in cells [57]. In a study, the cytotoxicity effect of nanodiamond particles was explored by correlating different surface functional groups on the nanoparticles, such as –OH, –COOH and –NH$_2$. It was shown that NDs were cytotoxic to HEK293 cells when the concentration was above 50 µg/mL. The cationic nanodiamond had the potential to permeate negatively charged cell membrane and hence exhibited cytotoxicity. In addition, carboxylated nanodiamond (ND–COOH) was reported to possess embryotoxicity as well as teratogenicity [58].

The in vitro toxicity effect of CBNPs (260 ± 13.7 nm) was evaluated on A549 human alveolar basal epithelial cells and suggested that ultrafine particles induced a greater oxidative stress with prolonged inhibitory effects than fine particles [59]. Printex 90, a commercial name of carbon black nanoparticles with a diameter of 14 nm, exhibited an oxidative damage response in HepG2 cells at 25 mg/L, which was revealed from formamidopyrimidine DNA glycosylase (Fpg)-modified comet assay [60]. In another comet (Fpg) assay, it was discovered that an increased level of oxidized purines was observed when the nanoparticles were investigated in the FE1-MML Muta Mouse lung epithelial cell line. The mutant frequency was noticed in carbon black exposed cells following eight repeated 72 h incubations with a cumulative dose of 6 mg nanoparticles [61]. The western blot analysis exposed that ultrafine carbon black nanoparticles, at 30.7 µg/cm^2, stimulated proliferation of human primary bronchial epithelial cells through oxidative stress and epidermal growth factor-mediated signaling pathway [62]. The cytotoxic and genotoxic effects of CBNPs were investigated on the mouse macrophage cell line RAW 264.7. The particle size and specific surface area was 14 nm and 300 m^2/g, respectively. The data confirmed acentric chromosome fragments at all concentrations and there was a slight increase in micronuclei frequencies at 3 and 10 mg/L [63]. It was reported that CBNPs (100 µg/mL) could induce DNA single-strand breaks and induce AP-1 and NFκB DNA binding in A549 lung epithelial cell line after 3 h of exposure [64]. The toxicity measurements of CBNPs in THP-1 derived monocytes and macrophages exemplified that the nanoparticles supported endothelial activation and lipid accumulation in THP-1 derived macrophages. In addition, the nanoparticles influenced increased cytotoxicity, LDH levels and intracellular ROS production in a dose-dependent manner [65].

It was discovered that C60 fullerene of approximately 0.7 nm was less toxic than carbon black and diesel exhaust particles when FE1-MutaMouse lung epithelial cells were exposed to nanoparticles. The results of the comet assay revealed that C60 significantly increased the quantity of formamidopyrimidine-glycosylase sites (22%) and oxidized purines (5%), though the nanoparticles did not involve breaking DNA strands [66]. Genotoxic effects of C60 sized 0.7 nm were investigated by micronuclei test in the human lung cancer cell line (A549) at a concentration range of 0.02–200 µg/mL and increased micronuclei frequencies were observed in nanoparticles treated cells in a dose-dependent manner [67]. The genotoxic studies of colloidal C60 in human lymphocytes had shown genotoxicity at 2.2 µg/L, whereas the ethanolic solution of C60 had exhibited the same at 0.42 µg/L [68]. The polyhydroxylated C60 fullerenol presented a dose-dependent decrease in micronuclei frequency and chromosome aberration when the nanoparticles were treated with Chinese hamster ovary cells (CHO K1). However, the study did not show any genotoxic effects in the concentrations of 11–221 µm [27]. The cytotoxicity of hydroxylated fullerene was analyzed in vascular endothelial cells at different concentrations, 1–100 µg/mL, and a dose-dependent decrease in cell viability was perceived. Furthermore, it was reported that fullerenes affected cell growth and cell attachment with the potential to cause cardiovascular disease after a long period of exposure (10 days) [69].

The toxicity effect of SWCNTs was explored on human embryonic kidney cells (HEK293T) and reported that the nanoparticle exposure resulted in a decrease in cell adhesion, inhibition in cell proliferation and induction in apoptosis, depending on the dosage and time. In addition, a nodular structure was formed due to the nanoparticle aggregation and overlap of cells [70]. The agglomeration of CNTs had a larger impact on triggering cellular toxicity in human MSTO-211H cells. It was found that the agglomerated CNTs were more toxic compared to monodispersed CNTs [71]. The geometric structure of the nanoparticles played a pivotal role in determining cytotoxicity. A comparative study was provided in describing cytotoxicity of SWCNTs, MWCNTs, and C60 fullerenes on guinea pig alveolar macrophages. The order of displaying toxicity was as follows, SWCNTs > MWCNTs > C60 fullerenes [72]. The intracellular distribution of functionalized SWCNTs was studied in murine 3T3 and human 3T6 fibroblast cells. The length of the nanotube varied from 300 to 1000 nm and the outer diameter was 1 nm. The analyses revealed that SWCNTs resided either in the cytoplasm or nucleus after crossing the cell membrane, and exhibited toxicity when the concentration of nanoparticles reached above 10 µM [73]. It was confirmed that exposure of SWCNTs induced cutaneous and pulmonary toxicities in human bronchial epithelial cells (BEAS-2B) and human keratinocyte cells (HaCaT). The microarray analysis revealed that the nanoparticles triggered alteration of genes followed by transcriptional responses. Cellular morphology, integrity and ultrastructure were affected as the nanoparticles depleted antioxidants in the cells [74,75]. Functionalization of the nanoparticles had taken advantage of reducing the toxic level of nanoparticles. The derivatized SWCNTs were reported to have fewer toxic effects than pristine SWCNTs from in vitro cytotoxicity measurements in human dermal fibroblasts [76]. The introduction of SWCNTs into normal and malignant human mesothelial cells produced ROS causing cell death, DNA damage and H2AX phosphorylation [77]. It was reported that SWCNTs, with a primary particle size of 0.4–1.2 nm and specific surface area of 26 m^2/g, had the potential to induce DNA damage in lung V79 fibroblasts [78].

The cytotoxic and genotoxic effects of single and multi-walled CNTs were studied on the mouse macrophage cell line RAW 264.7, and it was demonstrated that the exposure of nanoparticles stimulated ROS release, chromosomal aberrations, necrosis, and apoptosis, but they did not cause any inflammatory responses. In addition, MWCNTs were reported to penetrate the cell membrane and reside in the nuclear envelope [63]. Electron microscopic studies indicated that highly purified MWCNTs expressed higher cytotoxic effects by damaging the plasma membrane of mouse macrophages (J774.1). It was found that the cytotoxicity of MWCNTs was significantly larger than crocidolite, a fibrous form of sodium iron silicate [79]. The higher concentrated MWCNTs caused a decrease in cellular viability and an increase in inflammation on prolonged exposure to human epidermal keratinocytes (HEK) cells. The nanoparticles had the potential to penetrate the cell membrane and change the expression level of various proteins. The nanoparticles were reported to be abundantly present within cytoplasmic vacuoles of the cells after cell permeation [80]. The toxicity of MWCNTs of approximately 30 nm was evaluated in human skin fibroblasts (HSF42) and the results revealed that the nanoparticles disrupted intracellular signaling pathways, causing an increase in apoptosis and necrosis, and activated the genes associated with cellular cycle regulation, metabolism, cellular transport, and stress response [81]. Interestingly, oxidized MWCNTs were described to exhibit more toxicity than pristine MWCNTs. Both were reported to induce apoptosis in T lymphocytes depending on the time period and dose [82].

Table 1. The in Vitro Toxicity Effects of 0-D and 1-D Carbon Nanomaterials.

Carbon Nanomaterial; Nanoparticle Dimension	Cell Line; Concentrations; Exposure	Toxicity Effects	Reference
PEI-CQDs; PS = 6.5 ± 2 nm, HD = 56.54 nm	Kidney epithelial cells (African green monkey); 200, 400, 600 and 800 µg/mL; 48 h	PEI-CQDs exhibited toxic effects above concentration 600 µg/mL.	[46]
CQDs; PS = ~7 nm, HD = 60.3 ± 7 nm	Human bronchial epithelial cells (16HBE); 1, 10, 50, 100 and 200 µg/mL; 24 h	CQDs reduced cell viability inducing oxidative stress.	[47]
OH-GQDs; PS = 5.6 ± 1.1 nm, HD = 10.3 ± 1.9 nm	Human lung carcinoma cell lines (H1299 and A549); 12.5, 25, 50 and 100 µg/mL; 24 and 48 h	The hydroxylated GQDs induced cell senescence and inhibited Rb phosphorylation in both types of cells at concentration 50 µg/mL.	[50]
GQDs; PS = ~20 nm	Human breast cancer cells (MCF-7) and human gastric cancer cells (MGC-803); 20, 100, 200 and 400 µg/mL; 24 h	GQDs were found less cytotoxic on both type of cells though the nanoparticles permeated into cytoplasm and nucleus.	[51]
NDs; PS = 4–5 nm	Mouse embryonic stem cells; 5 or 100 µg/mL; 24 h	NDs exhibited genotoxicity, expressing an increased level of DNA repair proteins.	[52]
NDs; HD = 41–103 nm	Human keratinocyte (HaCaT) and human alveolar basal epithelial cells (A549); 0.01, 0.1 and 1.0 mg/mL; 6 and 24 h	NDs were not involved in decreasing cell viability and generating intracellular ROS. However, the nanoparticles inhibited colony formation in cells even at concentration 1.0 mg/mL.	[53]
NDs; PS = 6–500 nm	Mouse macrophages (RAW 264.7); 0, 10, 50, 100 and 200 µg/mL; 24 h	The results revealed that NDs reduced cell proliferation and metabolic activity in a dose dependent manner.	[54]
CBNPs; PS = 260 ± 13.7 nm	A549 cells; 0.39 and 0.78 µg/mL; 24 and 48 h	Size dependent cytotoxicity was observed in CBNPs treated cells. Ultrafine CBNPs affected more oxidative stress in cells than fine CBNPs.	[59]
CBNPs; PS = 14 nm	FE1-Muta mouse lung epithelial cell line; 75 µg/mL; 8 × 72 h	CBNPs caused genetic mutation increasing the quantity of oxidized purines.	[61]
CBNPs; PS = 14 nm, SSA = 300 m^2/g	RAW 264.7 cells; 0.25, 10, 25, 50 and 100 µg/mL; 24, 48 and 72 h	Cytotoxic and genotoxic effects were observed, along with the formation of acentric chromosome fragments at all concentrations.	[63]
CBNPs; PS = 14 nm	A549 cells; 100 µg/mL; 0.5–24 h	CBNPs induced DNA single-strand breaks at 100 µg/mL at 3 h of post exposure.	[64]

Table 1. Cont.

Carbon Nanomaterial; Nanoparticle Dimension	Cell Line; Concentrations; Exposure	Toxicity Effects	Reference
C60; PS = 0.7 nm	FE1-Muta mouse lung epithelial cells; 100 µg/mL; 576 h	C60 increased the level of oxidized purines significantly without affecting DNA strands.	[66]
C60; PS = 0.7 nm	A549 cells; 0.02–200 µg/mL; 48 h	C60 treated cells witnessed increased micronuclei frequency depending on dosage.	[67]
C60(OH)n	Chinese hamster ovary cells (CHO K1); 11–221 µM; 24 h	The nanoparticles treated cells showed decreased micronuclei frequency and chromosome aberration in a dose dependent manner.	[27]
C60(OH)n; PS = 7.1 ± 2.4 nm	Human umbilical vascular endothelial cells; 1–100 µg/mL; 24 h	The hydroxylated C60 decreased cell viability in a concentration dependent manner.	[69]
SWCNTs; n/a	Human embryonic kidney cells (HEK293T); 0.78, 1.56, 3.12, 6.25, 12.5, 25, 50, 100, 150 and 200 µg/mL; 0–5 days	SWCNTs decreased cell adhesion and inhibited cell proliferation depending on dose and time.	[70]
SWCNTs; L = 300–1000 nm, W = 1 nm	Murine 3T3 and human 3T6 fibroblast cells; 1, 5 and 10 µM; 1 h	The nanoparticles had the potential to permeate the cell and exhibited toxicity above 10 µM.	[73]
SWCNTs; PS = 0.8–2.0 nm	Normal and malignant human mesothelial cells; 12.5, 25 and 125 µg/cm^2; 24 h	DNA damage, cell death, and ROS generation were observed in nanoparticles treated cells.	[77]
SWCNTs; PS = 0.4–1.2 nm, SSA = 1040 m^2/g	Chinese hamster lung V79 fibroblasts; 0, 24, 48 and 96 µg/cm^2; 3 and 24 h	SWCNTs caused DNA damage in cells at 24 h of post-exposure.	[78]
MWCNTs; PS = 67 nm, SSA = 26 m^2/g	Mouse macrophages (J774.1 and CHO-K1); 10–1000 µg/mL; 16–32 h	MWCNTs treated cells exhibited larger cytotoxicity than crocidolite treated cells.	[79]
MWCNTs; PS = 100 nm	Human epidermal keratinocytes (HEK) cells; 0.1, 0.2 and 0.4 mg/mL; 1, 2, 4, 8, 12, 24 and 48 h	MWCNTs penetrated the cell membrane and altered the gene expression level of various proteins.	[80]
MWCNTs; PS = 30 nm	Human skin fibroblasts (HSF42); 0.06, 0.6 and 6 µg/mL; 48 h	MWCNTs caused an increase in apoptosis and necrosis disrupting intracellular signaling pathways, cell metabolism and cellular transport.	[81]
MWCNTs; L = 1–5 µm, W = 20–40 nm	Human blood T lymphocytes; 10 ng/cell; 0, 24, 48, 72, 96 and 120 h	The oxidized form of MWCNTs exhibited more cytotoxicity than pristine MWCNTs. Both types of nanoparticles induced apoptosis in cells in a time and dose dependent manner.	[82]

Abbreviations: PS, particle size; HD, hydrodynamic diameter; SSA, specific surface area; L, length; W, width; n/a, not available.

3. In Vivo Toxicity of Zero-and One-Dimensional Carbon Nanomaterials

In some studies, the researchers performed in vivo animal studies of carbon nanomaterials after the careful evaluation of their in vitro toxicity measurements, and some of studies are listed in Table 2.

Table 2. The in Vivo Toxicity Effects of 0-D and 1-D Carbon Nanomaterials.

Carbon Nanomaterial; Nanoparticle Dimension	Animal Model; Concentrations; Exposure	Toxicity Effects	Reference
CQDs; PS ≤ 10 nm, HD = 40 nm, IS = 0.32 nm	Zebrafish; 0, 10, 30, 50, 70, 100 and 200 mg/L; 0, 24, 48, 72, and 96 h Zooplankton; 0, 10, 30, 50, 70, 100 and 200 mg/L; 48 h Phytoplankton; 0, 5, 10, 50, 100, 200 and 500 mg/L; 0, 24, 48, 72, and 96 h	CQDs, at higher dose of 200 mg/L, did not affect swimming and feeding behaviors. CQDs exhibited moderate toxicity to zooplankton, inducing mortality and immobility with EC50 value 97.5 mg/L. CQDs induced oxidative stress and water acidification, inhibited photosynthesis and depleted nutrition absorption in a dose and time dependent manner. It retarded the growth of phytoplankton with EC50 value 74.8 mg/L at 96 h of the study.	[83]
CQDs; PS = 1–5 nm	Male and female ICR mice; 250, 320, 400 and 500 mg/kg, single dose, intravenous injections; 14 day sMale ICR mice; 100 mg/kg, repeated dose, intravenous injections; 1, 7, 30 and 90 days, once/day	Male mice (LD50 391.62 mg/kg) were found to be more sensitive to the higher doses of the nanoparticles than female mice (LD50 357.77 mg/kg). An acute inflammatory response was observed after seven doses, however the data on the body weight, organ coefficients, blood biochemistry, and organ histopathology suggested that the nanoparticles had low toxicity during the entire experimental period.	[84]
CQDs; PS = 2–6 nm	Male and female embryos/larvae of rare minnows; 0, 1, 5, 10, 20, 40, and 80 mg/L; 12–96 hpf	In lower dose treated groups (1, 5, 10, and 20 mg/L), no significant developmental defects were observed at the stage of 12 hpf, whereas higher dose treated groups (40 mg/L and 80 mg/L) caused embryos yolk agglutination in a concentration-dependent manner. The noticeable time-dependent deleterious effects were decreased spontaneous movements, higher heart rate, and increased hatching rate. Most of the unhatched embryos died when the exposure time reached 96 hpf.	[9]
CQDs; PS = 8 ± 2 nm	Male ICR mice; 0, 6, 12 and 24 mg/kg, intraperitoneal injection; 30 days	The histopathological examination showed that no obvious toxic effects were triggered by CQDs on mice. However, NMR metabolomic profiles revealed that CQDs could affect cell membrane, immune system, and normal liver clearance.	[8]

Table 2. Cont.

Carbon Nanomaterial; Nanoparticle Dimension	Animal Model; Concentrations; Exposure	Toxicity Effects	Reference
GQDs; PS = 2.3–6.4 nm, IS = 0.36 nm, height = 0.6–3.5 nm, 1–3 layers	AB strains of wild-type zebrafish embryo/larva; 0, 12.5, 25, 50, 100 and 200 µg/mL; 4–120 hpf	The heart rate of treated animals was found to be decreased with a dose-dependent effect. The exposure of GQDs suggested that they might have little effect during the heart development stage of zebrafish embryos and larvae.	[85]
GQDs, PS = 3.315 ± 1.74 nm	AB strains of wild-type zebrafish embryo/larva; 0, 12.5, 25, 50, 100, and 200 µg/mL; 4–96 hpf	At low concentrations of GQDs, no significant toxicity was observed. When the concentration was above 50 µg/mL, GQDs disturbed the embryonic development. The hatching rate and heart rate were decrease, accompanied with an increase in mortality. At high concentration of GQDs (200 µg/mL), various embryonic malformations including pericardial edema, vitelline cyst, bent tail, and bent spine occurred.	[86]
PEG-GQDs; PS = 3–5 nm, height = 0.5–1 nm, 1–2 layers	Female BALB/c mice; 20 mg/kg, intraperitoneal injection, multiple doses; 2 weeks	PEG-GQDs exhibited no-toxicity effects because of nanoparticle encapsulation.	[87]
COOH-GQDs; PS = 3–6 nm	SD rats; 5 and 10 mg/kg, intravenous injection; 7 doses in 22 days with an interval of 2 days	The studies revealed that the GQDs were distributed in liver, spleen, lung, kidney, and tumor sites after injection, however there was no obvious organ damage at 21 days of post-administration. The serum biochemistry and complete blood count studies revealed that the GQDs did not cause any significant toxicity to the treated animals.	[88]
NDs; HD = ~120 nm	Wild type young Caenorhabditis elegans; 0.5 mg/mL, microinjection	The NDs were found in the distal gonad and oocytes at 30 min after injection. No detectable toxicity effects were found in brood size and longevity of the treated animal groups.	[89]
NDs; PS = 4 and 50 nm, IS = 0.202 nm	Male ICR mice; 1.0 mg/kg, intratracheal instillation; 1, 7, 14 and 28 days of post-exposure	At 1 day of post-exposure, both kinds of nanoparticles produced a temporary increase in lung index but there was no trace of lipid peroxidation in lung tissue. During the whole exposure period, the burden of nanoparticle in macrophages was observed and the number of nanoparticles decreased by time in alveolar.	[90]

Table 2. Cont.

Carbon Nanomaterial; Nanoparticle Dimension	Animal Model; Concentrations; Exposure	Toxicity Effects	Reference
NDs; PS = 2–10 nm and 40–100 nm	Male Kun Ming mice; intratracheal instillation; 0.8, 4 and 20 mg/kg; 3 days	A dose-dependent toxicity effect was observed in the lung tissue of mice at 3 days of post-exposure of both kinds of nanoparticles and the higher concentration treated mice (4 and 20 mg/kg) exhibited significant toxicity.	[13]
NDs-BSA; PS = ~100 nm	Zebrafish (AB strain) embryos/larvae; 1, 2, 5 mg/mL; 4–96 hpf	The different stages of zebrafish embryos exhibited similar development when compared to the control groups at a lower concentration of NDs (1 mg/mL). However, a higher concentration of NDs affected the zebrafish embryos at the Pharyngula stage. The medium concentrated NDs (2 and 5 mg/mL) caused fin curving of zebrafish larvae at the hatching stage.	[14]
CBNPs; PS = 14 nm	Female C57BL/6J mice, 10 mg/mouse, intratracheal instillation; 21 days	CBNPs did not exert any significant adverse clinical effects. However, the histopathological studies revealed that they decreased lung compliance inducing inflammation when administered along with bleomycin. They augmented the levels of CCL2, TGF-b1, KC, IL-6, and nitrotyrosine in mice on different days of exposure.	[91]
CBNPs; PS = 14 and 56 nm	Male ICR mice; 50 µg/body, intratracheal instillation; 1, 7 or 14 days	CBNPs of 14 nm aggravated porcine pancreatic elastase mediated pulmonary exposure on emphysematous lung injury at an early stage (day 1) and expressed more interleukin-b and keratinocyte-derived chemoattractant. CBNPs of 56 nm caused inflammation but did not induce porcine pancreatic elastase triggered pathophysiology in the lung.	[92]
CBNPs; PS = 14 nm, SSA = 295–338 m^2/g	Time mated C57BL/6BomTac mice, 42 mg/m^3, whole-body inhalation; 1 h/day on gestation days (GD) 8–18 days 11, 54 and 268 µg/animal, intratracheal instillation; 1 h/day, GD 7, 10, 15 and 18 days	The whole-body inhalation induced significant DNA strand breaks in the liver of mothers and their offspring, whereas the intratracheal instillation did not have that effect. However, gestation and lactation were not affected in both ways of administrations. The pulmonary inflammation in time mated mice was similar in both administrations for the medium dose of nanoparticles.	[17]

Table 2. Cont.

Carbon Nanomaterial; Nanoparticle Dimension	Animal Model; Concentrations; Exposure	Toxicity Effects	Reference
CBNPs; PS = 14 nm, SSA = 295–338 m^2/g	Female C57BL/6 mice; 162 µg/mouse, intratracheal instillation; 3 h, 1, 2, 3, 4, 5, 14 and 42 days	In the initial days of post-exposure, the worsening of pulmonary homeostasis occurred by the induction of oxidative stress, DNA strand breaks, cell cycle arrest, and cell death. Multiple chronic pulmonary inflammatory processes were the possible effects at the later points of post-exposure days.	[18]
CBNPs; GMD = 53 ± 1.57 nm	Male C57BL/6 mice; 12.5 µg/m^3, nasal inhalation; 4 h/day, 7 days	The histopathology analyses revealed that the inhalation of nanoparticles exacerbated lung inflammation expressing a significant level of interleukin-6, interferon-γ, and fibronectin in lung tissues.	[93]
PAH-CBNPs; PS = 14.2 ± 0.1 nm, SSA = 115 ± 3 m^2/g	Male Wistar rats (strain Crl: WI (Han)); 6 mg/m^3, nasal inhalation; 6 h/day, 2 weeks	A significant increase in polymorphonuclear granulocyte numbers was observed for the animals treated with CBNPs and PAH-CBNPs when compared to clean air control on day 1 post-exposure. PAH-CBNPs induced bronchioalveolar hyperplasia, whereas CBNPs caused very slight histological alterations on day 14 post-exposure. When compared to control, only PAH-CBNPs exhibited significant IL-6 mRNA expression and keratinocyte chemoattractant.	[94]
C60; PS = 33 nm, SSA = 104.6 m^2/g	Male Wistar rats; 0.33, 0.66 and 3.3 mg/kg, intratracheal instillation; 3 days, 1 week, 1, 3 and 6 months	No significant increase was observed in total cell count and in the expression of the cytokine-induced neutrophil chemoattractants CINC-1, -2αβ and -3 at a low dose of fullerene treated groups. The higher dose of fullerene treated rat group showed a significant increase in gene expression and total cell counts.	[95]
	Male Wistar rats; 0.12 ± 0.03 mg/m^3, whole-body inhalation; 4 weeks, 6 h/day, 5 days/week	There were no significant changes in total cell count in BALF and gene expression of CINC-1, -2αβ and -3 in lung tissue.	
C60; GMD = 96 nm, SSA = 0.92 m^2/g	Male Wistar rats; 0.12 mg/m^3, whole-body inhalation; 4 weeks 6h/day, 5 days/week	Gene expression profiles revealed that the major histocompatibility complex (MHC) mediated immunity and metalloendopeptidase activity were upregulated at 3 days and 1 month of post-exposure. Some upregulated genes were involved in oxidative stress, inflammation, and apoptosis. The nanoparticles were found in alveolar epithelial cells and engulfed by macrophages.	[96]

Table 2. Cont.

Carbon Nanomaterial; Nanoparticle Dimension	Animal Model; Concentrations; Exposure	Toxicity Effects	Reference
C60; HD = 234.1 ± 48.9 nm and 856.5 ± 119.2 nm	gpt delta transgenic mice; 0.2 mg/animal, single dose, intratracheal instillation; 3 hMultiple doses (4 times)	Mutant frequencies were significantly increased (2–3 fold) in the lungs of the nanoparticle treated group when compared to control. There was a slight number of A:T to T:A transversion in C60 treated animals, while no genetic transversion was observed in control groups.	[67]
C60; PS = 46.7 ± 18.6 nm	ICR male mice; 0.5, 1, 2 mg/kg, intratracheal instillation; 1, 7, 14 and 28 days	Increase in pro-inflammatory cytokines including TNF-α, IL-1 and IL-6 and increase in T-cell distribution were observed in C60 treated mice. The gene expression of MHC class 2 was greater than that of MHC class 1 (H2-T23).	[97]
C60; HD = 407–5117 nm	Female Fisher 344 rats; single oral intragastric administration; 0.064 and 64 mg/kg; 24 h	Only high dose of fullerene generated oxidative damage by expressing a high level of mRNA 8-oxoguanine DNA glycosylase (8-oxodG) in the lung.	[98]
C60; n/a	Sprague-Dawley male and female rats; 2000 mg/kg, oral exposure, single dose; 14 days	No acute oral toxicity and no deaths were reported.	[26]
C60(OH)n	BALB/c female mice; 0.02, 0.2, 2.0, 20 and 200 µg/animal, intratracheal instillation; 24 h	The BAL data indicated that only 200 µg treated mice showed increased neutrophil influx in the lungs causing inflammation, whereas other low concentration treated groups did not present any significant changes.	[99]
SWCNTs; L ≤ 1 µm, W = 0.9–1.7 nm	Female Fisher 344 rats; 0.064 and 64 mg/Kg, single dose, oral intragastric administration; 24 h	SWCNTs were reported to cause oxidatively damaged DNA in lung and liver by increasing the level of 8-oxodG.	[98]
SWCNTs; n/a	Male Sprague-Dawley rats; 0.4, 2 and 4 mg/kg, intrapulmonary instillation; 1, 7, 30 and 90 days	Increase in lung granulomatous and inflammatory responses along with fibrosis and collagen deposition was observed in a time and dose-dependent manner for SWCNTs treated groups.	[41]
SWCNTs; L = 10 nm to several µm, W = 1–2 nm	Male ICR mice; 0.5 mg/kg, intratracheal instillation, single dose; 3 and 14 days	The histological data of SWCNTs treated groups revealed that an increase in macrophage infiltration, foamy-like macrophages formation in the alveolar space, and no significant granuloma formation were observed at 3 days of investigation. Meanwhile, a profound multifocal granuloma was found after 14 days.	[40]

Table 2. Cont.

Carbon Nanomaterial; Nanoparticle Dimension	Animal Model; Concentrations; Exposure	Toxicity Effects	Reference
SWCNTs; n/a	Female C57BL/6 mice; 40 µg/mouse, single dose, intraperitoneal injection; 1 and 7 days	Non-degraded nanotubes treated mice induced inflammation and tissue granulomas, while biodegraded nanotubes treated mice were not induced.	[100]
SWCNTs; L ≤ 5 µm, W = ~8 nm	SPF male and female Wistar rats; 2 and 10 mg/kg, intratracheal instillation; 5 weeks	High dose exposure of SWCNTs registered increased level of inflammatory markers such as IL-1, IL-6 and TNF-α in BALF than low dose exposure in rat lungs. Transgelin 2 gene expression was also found to be higher in high dose treated rats.	[101]
SWCNTs; HD = 48.4 nm	Male ICR mice; 25, 50 and 100 µg/kg, intratracheal instillation; after 24 h	The administration of SWCNTs increased the secretion of IL-6 and MCP-1, and the number of total cells including neutrophils, lymphocytes, and eosinophils in the lungs of higher dose-treated mice.	[39]
SWCNTs; L = ≤1 µm, W = 0.8–1.7 nm	Female C57BL/6J mice; 0.9, 2.8, 8.4 mg/kg, intratracheal instillation, single dose; 1, 3 and 28 days	A dose-dependent increase in Saa3 mRNA expression was observed in the lung.	[102]
SWCNTs; PS = 1–2 nm, SSA = 1040 m^2/g	Female C57BL/6J mice; 40 µg/mouse, pharyngeal aspiration, single dose; 1, 7 and 28 days	The SWCNTs treated vitamin E-deficient mice had shown a greater decrease in pulmonary antioxidants when compared to controls. Acute inflammation and enhanced profibrotic responses were also observed.	[42]
SWCNTs; L = ≤1 µm, W = 0.8–1.2 nm, SSA = 400–1000 m^2/g	Male C57BL/6J mice; 10 µg/mouse, pharyngeal aspiration, single dose; 2 weeks	Both Survanta (natural lung surfactant) dispersed and acetone/sonication dispersed SWCNTs induced lung fibrosis in mice by increasing collagen deposition.	[43]
MWCNTs; PS = 15–50 nm	Male Wistar rats; 5mg/m^3, nasal inhalation; single dose; 4 h, 1, 7, and 14 days	A significant increase in cell count, lactate dehydrogenase, alkaline phosphatase, and cytokines and a decrease in cell viability and alveolar macrophage count were observed in MWCNTs-treated rats in all the investigated days, when compared to control rats. Inflammation, granuloma, and fibrosis were also reported in the lungs of MWCNTs-treated rats on 7 and 14 days of post-exposure.	[32]

Table 2. Cont.

Carbon Nanomaterial; Nanoparticle Dimension	Animal Model; Concentrations; Exposure	Toxicity Effects	Reference
MWCNTs; short (L = 1–5 µm, W = 15 ± 5 nm), intermediate (L = 5–20 µm, W = 15 ± 5 nm), long (L = ~13 µm, W = 40–50 nm)	Female C57Bl/6 mice; 50 mg/mouse, intraperitoneal injection; 1 and 7 days	Size-dependent studies revealed that long sized MWCNTs (mean 13 µm) affected significant inflammation and granuloma in mice at 1 and 7 days of post-operation while short (1–5 µm) and intermediate (5–20 µm) MWCNTs did not cause any significant changes. Furthermore, short MWCNTs were readily involved in phagocytosis while long sized MWCNTs had frustrated phagocytosis.	[103]
MWCNTs; L = 1.1 ± 2.7 µm, W = 63 ± 1.5 nm	Male Wistar rats; 0.66 and 3.3 mg/kg, intratracheal instillation; 3, 7, 30, 90, and 180 days Male Wistar rats; whole-body inhalation; 6 h/day, 4 weeks	Lung inflammations and CINC-1 expressions were found significantly in high dose treated rats and temporary inflammation was observed in the low dose treated groups. Minimal pulmonary inflammation and a temporary increase in CINC-1 to CINC-3 expressions were found.	[104]
MWCNTs; L = 5.9 ± 0.05 µm, W = 9.7 ± 2.1 nm, SSA = 378 ± 20 m^2/g	Female Sprague–Dawley rats; 0.5 and 2 mg/rat, intratracheal instillation; 0, 28 and 60 days	At 60 days, pulmonary lesions were observed for MWCNTs treated rats owing to collagen-rich granulomas formation protruding in the bronchial lumen. TNF-α was excessively produced in the lungs of treated animals.	[105]
MWCNTs; n/a	Male guinea pigs; 12.5 mg/pig, intratracheal instillation; 90 days	At 90 days, the MWCNTs exposure caused pneumonitis with mild peribronchiolar fibrosis in pigs, which was not observed in the controls.	[106]

Abbreviations: PS, particle size; IS, interlayer spacing; HD, hydrodynamic diameter; GMD, geometric mean diameter; SSA, specific surface area; L, length; W, width; n/a, not available.

The toxicity of carbon quantum dots was investigated in different species such as zebrafish, zooplankton, and phytoplankton. The primary particle size was less than 10 nm, with interlayer spacing of 0.32 nm. It was found that zooplankton was more sensitive to CQDs than zebrafish and phytoplankton species and suffered oxidative stress, water acidification, insufficiency of nutrients and no photosynthesis in a time and dose-dependent manner [83]. When the nanoparticles were administered intravenously to ICR male and female mice with a single dose, it was observed that male mice are more sensitive than female mice, and that the nanoparticles treated male mice suffered severe acute inflammatory responses [84]. The intraperitoneal injection of CQDs (8 ± 2 nm) into male ICR mice affected cell membrane, immune system and liver clearance rate [8]. While investigating the in vivo toxicity of CQDs (2–6 nm) in embryos/larvae of male and female rare minnow, concentration-dependent embryos yolk agglutination, decreased spontaneous movements, and increased heart rate were observed [9]. The toxicity studies of GQDs in AB strains of wild-type zebrafish embryos/larvae revealed that the nanoparticle had the potential to decrease heart rate, causing disrupted embryonic development in a concentration dependent manner. However, the treatment of nanoparticles did not have significant toxicity at lower doses [85,86]. The toxicity of functional GQDs in an animal model was studied to understand the influence of functional groups attached on the surface of nanoparticles. The polyethylene glycol modified GQDs (PEG-GQDs) exhibited no significant toxicity when the nanoparticles were instilled intraperitoneally into female BALB/c mice [87]. Likewise, carboxylated GQDs (COOH-GQDs) triggered no obvious damage to SD rats after 21 days of intravenous post-administration [88].

The microinjection of NDs (0.5 mg/mL) to wild type young Caenorhabditis elegans had shown no detectable toxicity in brood size and longevity of animals. The hydrodynamic diameter of the nanoparticles in solution was approximately 120 nm [89]. When NDs of approximately 4 nm were intratracheally injected into male ICR mice at a concentration of 1.0 mg/kg, the nanoparticles produced lung burden during the whole exposure time, but there was no event of lipid peroxidation in lung tissue [90]. A dose-dependent toxicity was observed in the lung tissue of male Kun Ming mice after the NDs were intratracheally administered at different concentrations 0.8, 4.0 and 20 mg/kg [13]. While investigating possible toxicity of bovine serum albumin functionalized nanodiamond (ND-BSA, ~100 nm) in AB strain zebrafish embryos at a concentration range of 1–5 mg/mL and 4–96 h post-fertilization (hpf), it was found that the control and NDs treated groups had no significant differences in embryonic development at concentration of 1 mg/mL. However, a higher concentration of NDs affected the pharyngula stage of embryos and caused fin curve in larvae during the hatching stage [14].

There were many reports that demonstrated the toxicity of carbon nanomaterials in animal models, which included pulmonary inflammation, DNA breaks, oxidative stress and elevated expression of mRNAs [17,91–106]. The intratracheally administered CBNPs (67 μg/animal) to female pregnant mice did not trigger significant germline mutation when compared to the control [107]. When the rats were exposed to 7.1 and 52.8 mg/m^3 of CBNPs for 13 weeks, a significant dose-dependent increase in hypoxanthine-guanine phosphoribosyltransferase (hprt) mutation frequency was observed in rat alveolar epithelial cells. The nanoparticles impaired lung clearance, causing lung burden, and changed the expression of bronchoalveolar lavage fluid (BALF) markers of inflammation and lung injury [108]. Various immunohistochemical measurements were established to quantify DNA damage markers such as poly (ADP-ribose), 8-hydroxyguanosine, and 8-oxoguanine DNA glycosylase after intratracheally instilling CBNPs into rats for 3 months. The analyses revealed that the nanoparticles had significantly increased the expression of DNA damage markers, though the genotoxicity was less pronounced [109]. Genotoxic effects, acute phase and inflammatory responses were examined while exposing C57BL/6JBomTac mice to CBNPs. Even at low exposure doses of nanoparticles (0.67, 2, 6 μg), an increase in DNA strand breaks occurred in bronchoalveolar lavage (BAL) cells. It was reported that DNA damage was triggered by primary genotoxicity without inflammatory responses [110]. The pulmonary toxicity of carbon black nanoparticles was studied in C57BL/6 female mice administering a single dose of 0.162 mg. An increase in expression of miRNAs such as miR-135b, miR-21, and miR-146b, which are associated with pulmonary inflammation, was observed [111]. The polycyclic aromatic hydrocarbon modified CBNPs (PAH-CBNPs) were demonstrated to express the noticeable amount of keratinocyte chemoattractant and IL-6 mRNA, when compared to uncoated CBNPs and air control when male Wistar rats were subjected to nasal inhalation exposure for 2 weeks at a concentration of 6 mg/m^3. The primary particle size and specific surface area of functionalized CBNPs was 14.2 ± 0.1 and 115 ± 3 m^2/g, respectively [94].

The toxicity of fullerene of 96 nm was studied after subjecting male Wistar rats to whole-body inhalation for 4 weeks. The experiment was carried out for 6h/day with the exposure of 0.12 mg/m^3. No significant changes were reported in the gene expression of CINC-1, CINC-2αβ, and CINC-3 in lung tissue [95]. In another similar study, the upregulation of genes associated with inflammation, oxidative stress and apoptosis was noted after one month of nanoparticle exposure. The geometric mean diameter of fullerene nanoparticles was 96 nm and specific surface area of them was 0.92 m^2/g [96]. The intratracheal instillation of C60 to gpt delta transgenic mice at a single dose of 0.2 mg/mouse induced mutant frequencies with 2–3-fold increase in comparison to the control. When administered at multiple doses (4 times), the nanoparticles brought about transversion of A:T to T:A in treated animals [67]. The intratracheally instilled C60 (46.7 ± 18.6 nm) increased the expression of pro-inflammatory cytokines including tumor necrosis factor-α (TNF-α), interleukins (IL-1 and IL-6) and T-cell distribution in ICR male mice [97]. It was demonstrated that single oral intragastric administration of fullerene to female Fisher 344 rats generated oxidative damage along with the expression of mRNA 8-oxoguanine DNA glycosylase (8-oxodG) in the lung at high dose [98]. No acute oral toxicity was reported for the C60 treated Sprague-Dawley male and female rats for 2 weeks [26]. The intratracheally administered fullerenol (C60(OH)$_n$) showed increased neutrophil influx in the lungs causing inflammation in BALB/c female mice after 24 h of post-administration of 200 µg/mouse [99].

The DNA damage was examined in rats following intragastric instillation of SWCNT at a concentration of 0.64 mg/kg body weight. SWCNTs were demonstrated to elevate the levels of 8-oxodG in liver and lung tissues of rats. The length and width of the nanoparticles was less than 1 µm and 0.9–1.7 nm, respectively [98]. The aortic mitochondrial alteration was studied using oxidative stress assays in SWCNTs exposed C57BL/6 mice. The intra-pharyngeal instilled SWCNTs (40 µg/mouse) activated heme oxygenase 1, which is indicative of oxidative stress. The nanoparticles exhibited increased mitochondrial DNA damage accompanied by the changes in aortic mitochondrial protein carbonyl and glutathione levels [112].

The general toxicity effects of MWCNTs were inflammation, granuloma and fibrosis when in vivo toxicity measurements were performed in experimental animals [103,104,106]. The induction of mesothelioma in p53+/− mouse was studied by the intraperitoneal application of multi-wall carbon nanotube. It was found that intraperitoneally administered, micro-sized MWCNTs (10–20 µm) stimulated mesothelioma such as the positive control, crocidolite [113]. The immune and inflammatory responses of MWCNTs were tested following intraperitoneal administration of a single dose of 2 mg/kg body weight to female ICR mice. After 1 week of post-exposure, the expression of leukocyte adhesion molecules and cluster of differentiation on granulocytes were found increased. The number of monocytes, leukocytes, and granulocytes were also present in peripheral blood significantly. MWCNTs were reported to exhibit sustained immune responses with the overexpressed ovalbumin specific IgG1 and IgM. The original morphology of the liver had also suffered changes to a rounded shape along with the appearance of MWCNTs on internal organs [114].

4. Conclusions and Perspectives

In this review, we have discussed the toxicity effects of 0-D and 1-D carbon nanomaterials in different cell lines and animal models. It was demonstrated that differential toxicity of carbon nanomaterials was inherited from various factors such as size, dispersion, cell permeability, and functionalization. Though the researchers studied the toxicity of carbon nanomaterials in both in vitro and in vivo intensively, there are still some issues to be addressed. (1) Many researchers showed experimental results with the aim of comparing the toxicity of two or more carbon-based nanoparticles for the same cell line and animal model. A comparative study is required for different cell line sources and animal species for the same kind of nanoparticle. (2) There are many studies that emphasize the role of the encapsulating agents on the nanoparticles in altering the overall functionality. The differential toxicity depending on the charge on the surface of nanoparticles has also been demonstrated. However, a systematic study is needed to corroborate the toxicity results with the surface charge of the nanoparticles (either positive or negative) with subtle differences. (3) The toxicity studies of the same kind of carbon nanoparticle prepared from different techniques should also be examined. The following suggestions are put forth for future research in this field: (1) A comprehensive study on the toxicity of carbon nanomaterials using different physicochemical and biological parameters to exemplify toxicity limitation and prove the effectiveness of the materials. (2) A systematic study to ensure that the carbon nanoparticles exhibit toxicity towards cancerous cells but not normal cells at the established concentration range. Undoubtedly, the knowledge of the toxicity of carbon nanomaterials will help the researchers with interdisciplinary backgrounds to deliver more successful biocompatible materials to society in the future.

Author Contributions: I.-S.R. and D.-W.H. developed the idea and structure of the review article. I.S.R. and S.J.S. wrote the paper using the materials supplied by M.S.K., Y.B.L., B.K., S.W.H., and S.J.J., J.-C.L. revised and improved the manuscript. D.W.H. supervised the manuscript. All the authors have given approval to the final version of the manuscript.

Funding: This research was supported by the Bio & Medical Technology Development Program of the National Research Foundation (NRF) funded by the Korean government (MEST, No. 2015M3A9E2028643), Ministry of Trade, Industry and Energy (MOTIE, Korea, No. N0002310 and Technology Innovation Program No. 20000397), and Korea Research Institute of Chemical Technology (KRICT, Daejeon and Ulsan, Korea) and Ulsan City (SI1941-20, BS.K19-251).

Conflicts of Interest: The authors declare no conflict of interest.

References

1. Raza, M.A.; Kanwal, Z.; Rauf, A.; Sabri, A.N.; Riaz, S.; Naseem, S. Size- and Shape-Dependent Antibacterial Studies of Silver Nanoparticles Synthesized by Wet Chemical Routes. *Nanomaterials* **2016**, *6*, 74. [CrossRef]
2. Han, X.; Li, S.; Peng, Z.; Al-Yuobi, A.O.; Bashammakh, A.S.O.; El-Shahawi, M.S.; Leblanc, R.M. Interactions between Carbon Nanomaterials and Biomolecules. *J. Oleo Sci.* **2016**, *65*, 1–7. [CrossRef]
3. Cacciotti, I.; Chronopoulou, L.; Palocci, C.; Amalfitano, A.; Cantiani, M.; Cordaro, M.; Lajolo, C.; Callà, C.; Boninsegna, A.; Lucchetti, D.; et al. Controlled release of 18-β-glycyrrhetic acid by nanodelivery systems increases cytotoxicity on oral carcinoma cell line. *Nanotechnology* **2018**, *29*, 285101. [CrossRef]
4. Ramos, A.P.; Cruz, M.A.E.; Tovani, C.B.; Ciancaglini, P. Biomedical applications of nanotechnology. *Biophys. Rev.* **2017**, *9*, 79–89. [CrossRef]
5. Reddy, L.H.; Arias, J.L.; Nicolas, J.; Couvreur, P. Magnetic Nanoparticles: Design and Characterization, Toxicity and Biocompatibility, Pharmaceutical and Biomedical Applications. *Chem. Rev.* **2012**, *112*, 5818–5878. [CrossRef]
6. Zhu, S.; Gong, L.; Xie, J.; Gu, Z.; Zhao, Y. Design, Synthesis, and Surface Modification of Materials Based on Transition-Metal Dichalcogenides for Biomedical Applications. *Small Methods* **2017**, *1*, 1700220. [CrossRef]
7. Cha, C.; Shin, S.R.; Annabi, N.; Dokmeci, M.R.; Khademhosseini, A. Carbon-Based Nanomaterials: Multifunctional Materials for Biomedical Engineering. *ACS Nano* **2013**, *7*, 2891–2897. [CrossRef]
8. Hong, W.; Liu, Y.; Li, M.H.; Xing, Y.X.; Chen, T.; Fu, Y.H.; Jiang, L.; Zhao, H.; Jia, A.Q.; Wang, J.-S. In vivo toxicology of carbon dots by 1H NMR-based metabolomics. *Toxicol. Res.* **2018**, *7*, 834–847. [CrossRef]
9. Xiao, Y.Y.; Liu, L.; Chen, Y.; Zeng, Y.L.; Liu, M.Z.; Jin, L. Developmental Toxicity of Carbon Quantum Dots to the Embryos/Larvae of Rare Minnow (*Gobiocypris rarus*). *BioMed Res. Int.* **2016**, *2016*, 1–11. [CrossRef]
10. Xu, Y.; Tang, C.J.; Huang, H.; Sun, C.Q.; Zhang, Y.K.; Ye, Q.F.; Wang, A.J. Green Synthesis of Fluorescent Carbon Quantum Dots for Detection of Hg^{2+}. *Chin. J. Anal. Chem.* **2014**, *42*, 1252–1258. [CrossRef]
11. Cayuela, A.; Soriano, M.L.; Carrion, C.C.; Valcárcel, M. Semiconductor and carbon-based fluorescent nanodots: The need for consistency. *Chem. Commun.* **2016**, *52*, 1311–1326. [CrossRef] [PubMed]
12. Cole, I.S.; Wang, D.S.; Li, Q. The toxicity of graphene quantum dots. *RSC Adv.* **2016**, *6*, 89867–89878.
13. Zhang, X.; Yin, J.; Kang, C.; Li, J.; Zhu, Y.; Li, W.; Huang, Q.; Zhu, Z. Biodistribution and toxicity of nanodiamonds in mice after intratracheal instillation. *Toxicol. Lett.* **2010**, *198*, 237–243. [CrossRef] [PubMed]
14. Lin, Y.C.; Wu, K.T.; Lin, Z.R.; Perevedentseva, E.; Karmenyan, A.; Lin, M.D.; Cheng, C.L.; Lin, Y.; Wu, K.; Cheng, C. Nanodiamond for biolabelling and toxicity evaluation in the zebrafish embryo in vivo. *J. Biophotonics* **2016**, *9*, 827–836. [CrossRef]
15. Silbajoris, R.; Linak, W.; Shenderova, O.; Winterrowd, C.; Chang, H.-C.; Zweier, J.L.; Kota, A.; Dailey, L.A.; Nunn, N.; Bromberg, P.A.; et al. Detonation nanodiamond toxicity in human airway epithelial cells is modulated by air oxidation. *Diam. Relat. Mater.* **2015**, *58*, 16–23. [CrossRef]
16. Chaudhuri, I.; Fruijtier-Polloth, C.; Ngiewih, Y.; Levy, L. Evaluating the evidence on genotoxicity and reproductive toxicity of carbon black: A critical review. *Crit. Rev. Toxicol.* **2018**, *48*, 143–169. [CrossRef]
17. Jackson, P.; Hougaard, K.S.; Boisen, A.M.Z.; Jacobsen, N.R.; Jensen, K.A.; Møller, P.; Brunborg, G.; Gützkow, K.B.; Andersen, O.; Loft, S.; et al. Pulmonary exposure to carbon black by inhalation or instillation in pregnant mice: Effects on liver DNA strand breaks in dams and offspring. *Nanotoxicology* **2012**, *6*, 486–500. [CrossRef] [PubMed]

18. Husain, M.; Kyjovska, Z.O.; Bourdon-Lacombe, J.; Saber, A.T.; Jensen, K.A.; Jacobsen, N.R.; Williams, A.; Wallin, H.; Halappanavar, S.; Vogel, U.; et al. Carbon black nanoparticles induce biphasic gene expression changes associated with inflammatory responses in the lungs of C57BL/6 mice following a single intratracheal instillation. *Toxicol. Appl. Pharmacol.* **2015**, *289*, 573–588. [CrossRef]
19. Gray, C.A.; Muranko, H. Studies of Robustness of Industrial Aciniform Aggregates and Agglomerates—Carbon Black and Amorphous Silicas: A Review Amplified by New Data. *J. Occup. Environ. Med.* **2006**, *48*, 1279–1290. [CrossRef]
20. Watson, A.Y.; Valberg, P.A. Carbon Black and Soot: Two Different Substances. *AIHA J.* **2001**, *62*, 218–228. [CrossRef]
21. Zhang, W.; Liu, Q.; Chen, P. Flexible Strain Sensor Based on Carbon Black/Silver Nanoparticles Composite for Human Motion Detection. *Materials* **2018**, *11*, 1836. [CrossRef]
22. Mazzaracchio, V.; Tomei, M.R.; Cacciotti, I.; Chiodoni, A.; Novara, C.; Castellino, M.; Scordo, G.; Amine, A.; Moscone, D.; Arduini, F. Inside the different types of carbon black as nanomodifiers for screen-printed electrodes. *Electrochim. Acta* **2019**, *317*, 673–683. [CrossRef]
23. Johnston, H.J.; Hutchison, G.R.; Christensen, F.M.; Aschberger, K.; Stone, V. The biological mechanisms and physicochemical characteristics responsible for driving fullerene toxicity. *Toxicol. Sci.* **2010**, *114*, 162–182. [CrossRef]
24. Nielsen, G.D.; Roursgaard, M.; Jensen, K.A.; Poulsen, S.S.; Larsen, S.T. In vivoBiology and Toxicology of Fullerenes and Their Derivatives. *Basic Clin. Pharmacol. Toxicol.* **2008**, *103*, 197–208. [CrossRef]
25. Aschberger, K.; Johnston, H.J.; Stone, V.; Aitken, R.J.; Tran, C.L.; Hankin, S.M.; Peters, S.A.; Christensen, F.M. Review of fullerene toxicity and exposure—Appraisal of a human health risk assessment, based on open literature. *Regul. Toxicol. Pharmacol.* **2010**, *58*, 455–473. [CrossRef]
26. Mori, T.; Takada, H.; Ito, S.; Matsubayashi, K.; Miwa, N.; Sawaguchi, T. Preclinical studies on safety of fullerene upon acute oral administration and evaluation for no mutagenesis. *Toxicology* **2006**, *225*, 48–54. [CrossRef]
27. Mrđanović, J.; Solajic, S.; Bogdanovic, V.; Stankov, K.; Bogdanovic, G.; Djordjevic, A. Effects of fullerenol $C_{60}(OH)_{24}$ on the frequency of micronuclei and chromosome aberrations in CHO-K1 cells. *Mutat. Res. Toxicol. Environ. Mutagen.* **2009**, *680*, 25–30. [CrossRef]
28. Antunes, M.; Velasco, J.I. Multifunctional polymer foams with carbon nanoparticles. *Prog. Polym. Sci.* **2014**, *39*, 486–509. [CrossRef]
29. Tong, C.W.; Berawi, M.A.; Khalil, M.; Jan, B.M. Advanced nanomaterials in oil and gas industry: Design, application and challenges. *Appl. Energy* **2017**, *191*, 287–310.
30. Wu, D.; Wu, L.; Zhou, W.; Sun, Y.; Zhang, M. Relations between the aspect ratio of carbon nanotubes and the formation of percolation networks in biodegradable polylactide/carbon nanotube composites. *J. Polym. Sci. Part B Polym. Phys.* **2010**, *48*, 479–489. [CrossRef]
31. Ando, Y.; Zhao, X.; Sugai, T.; Kumar, M. Growing carbon nanotubes. *Mater. Today* **2004**, *7*, 22–29. [CrossRef]
32. Francis, A.P.; Ganapathy, S.; Palla, V.R.; Murthy, P.B.; Ramaprabhu, S.; Devasena, T. One time nose-only inhalation of MWCNTs: Exploring the mechanism of toxicity by intermittent sacrifice in Wistar rats. *Toxicol. Rep.* **2015**, *2*, 111–120. [CrossRef] [PubMed]
33. Kobayashi, N.; Izumi, H.; Morimoto, Y. Review of toxicity studies of carbon nanotubes. *J. Occup. Health* **2017**, *59*, 394–407. [CrossRef] [PubMed]
34. Ema, M.; Gamo, M.; Honda, K. A review of toxicity studies of single-walled carbon nanotubes in laboratory animals. *Regul. Toxicol. Pharmacol.* **2016**, *74*, 42–63. [CrossRef] [PubMed]
35. Mohanta, D.; Patnaik, S.; Sood, S.; Das, N. Carbon nanotubes: Evaluation of toxicity at biointerfaces. *J. Pharm. Anal.* **2019**. [CrossRef]
36. Singh, E.; Srivastava, R.; Kumar, U.; Katheria, A.D. Carbon nanotube: A review on introduction, fabrication techniques and optical applications. *Nanosci. Nanotechnol. Res.* **2017**, *4*, 120–126.
37. Vlasova, I.I.; Sokolov, A.V.; Chekanov, A.V.; Kostevich, V.A.; Vasilyev, V.B. Myeloperoxidase-induced biodegradation of single-walled carbon nanotubes is mediated by hypochlorite. *Russ. J. Bioorganic Chem.* **2011**, *37*, 453–463. [CrossRef]
38. Tasis, D.; Tagmatarchis, N.; Bianco, A.; Prato, M. Chemistry of Carbon Nanotubes. *Chem. Rev.* **2006**, *106*, 1105–1136. [CrossRef]

39. Park, E.J.; Zahari, N.E.M.; Kang, M.S.; Lee, S.J.; Lee, K.; Lee, B.S.; Yoon, C.; Cho, M.H.; Kim, Y.; Kim, J.H. Toxic response of HIPCO single-walled carbon nanotubes in mice and RAW264.7 macrophage cells. *Toxicol. Lett.* **2014**, *229*, 167–177. [CrossRef]
40. Chou, C.C.; Hsiao, H.Y.; Hong, Q.S.; Chen, C.H.; Peng, Y.W.; Chen, H.W.; Yang, P.C. Single-Walled Carbon Nanotubes Can Induce Pulmonary Injury in Mouse Model. *Nano Lett.* **2008**, *8*, 437–445. [CrossRef]
41. Al Faraj, A.; Bessaad, A.; Cieślar, K.; Lacroix, G.; Canet-Soulas, E.; Crémillieux, Y. Long-term follow-up of lung biodistribution and effect of instilled SWCNTs using multiscale imaging techniques. *Nanotechnology* **2010**, *21*, 175103. [CrossRef] [PubMed]
42. Shvedova, A.A.; Kisin, E.R.; Murray, A.R.; Gorelik, O.; Arepalli, S.; Castranova, V.; Young, S.-H.; Gao, F.; Tyurina, Y.Y.; Oury, T.D.; et al. Vitamin E Deficiency Enhances Pulmonary Inflammatory Response and Oxidative Stress Induced by Single Walled Carbon Nanotubes in C57BL/6 Mice. *Toxicol. Appl. Pharmacol.* **2007**, *221*, 339–348. [CrossRef] [PubMed]
43. Wang, L.; Castranova, V.; Mishra, A.; Chen, B.; Mercer, R.R.; Schwegler-Berry, D.; Rojanasakul, Y. Dispersion of single-walled carbon nanotubes by a natural lung surfactant for pulmonary in vitro and in vivo toxicity studies. *Part. Fibre Toxicol.* **2010**, *7*, 31. [CrossRef] [PubMed]
44. Catalán, J.; Siivola, K.M.; Nymark, P.; Lindberg, H.K.; Suhonen, S.; Järventaus, H.; Koivisto, A.J.; Moreno, C.; Vanhala, E.; Wolff, H.; et al. In vitro and in vivo genotoxic effects of straight versus tangled multi-walled carbon nanotubes. *Nanotoxicology* **2016**, *10*, 1–47. [CrossRef] [PubMed]
45. Rittinghausen, S.; Hackbarth, A.; Creutzenberg, O.; Ernst, H.; Heinrich, U.; Leonhardt, A.; Schaudien, D. The carcinogenic effect of various multi-walled carbon nanotubes (MWCNTs) after intraperitoneal injection in rats. *Part. Fibre Toxicol.* **2014**, *11*, 59. [CrossRef] [PubMed]
46. Emam, A.N.; Loutfy, S.A.; Mostafa, A.A.; Awad, H.; Mohamed, M.B. Cyto-toxicity, biocompatibility and cellular response of carbon dots–plasmonic based nano-hybrids for bioimaging. *RSC Adv.* **2017**, *7*, 23502–23514. [CrossRef]
47. Zhang, X.; He, X.; Li, Y.; Zhang, Z.; Ma, Y.; Li, F.; Liu, J. A cytotoxicity study of fluorescent carbon nanodots using human bronchial epithelial cells. *J. Nanosci. Nanotechnol.* **2013**, *13*, 5254–5259. [CrossRef] [PubMed]
48. Havrdova, M.; Hola, K.; Skopalik, J.; Tomankova, K.; Petr, M.; Cepe, K.; Polakova, K.; Tucek, J.; Bourlinos, A.B.; Zboril, R. Toxicity of carbon dots—Effect of surface functionalization on the cell viability, reactive oxygen species generation and cell cycle. *Carbon* **2016**, *99*, 238–248. [CrossRef]
49. Zhu, S.; Zhang, J.; Qiao, C.; Tang, S.; Li, Y.; Yuan, W.; Li, B.; Tian, L.; Liu, F.; Hu, R.; et al. Strongly green-photoluminescent graphene quantum dots for bioimaging applications. *Chem. Commun.* **2011**, *47*, 6858–6860. [CrossRef] [PubMed]
50. Tian, X.; Xiao, B.-B.; Wu, A.; Yu, L.; Zhou, J.; Wang, Y.; Wang, N.; Guan, H.; Shang, Z.-F. Hydroxylated-graphene quantum dots induce cells senescence in both p53-dependent and -independent manner. *Toxicol. Res.* **2016**, *5*, 1639–1648. [CrossRef] [PubMed]
51. Wu, C.; Wang, C.; Han, T.; Zhou, X.; Guo, S.; Zhang, J. Insight into the Cellular Internalization and Cytotoxicity of Graphene Quantum Dots. *Adv. Health Mater.* **2013**, *2*, 1613–1619. [CrossRef] [PubMed]
52. Xing, Y.; Xiong, W.; Zhu, L.; Osawa, E.; Hussin, S.; Dai, L. DNA Damage in Embryonic Stem Cells Caused by Nanodiamonds. *ACS Nano* **2011**, *5*, 2376–2384. [CrossRef] [PubMed]
53. Horie, M.; Komaba, L.K.; Kato, H.; Nakamura, A.; Yamamoto, K.; Endoh, S.; Fujita, K.; Kinugasa, S.; Mizuno, K.; Hagihara, Y.; et al. Evaluation of cellular influences induced by stable nanodiamond dispersion; the cellular influences of nanodiamond are small. *Diam. Relat. Mater.* **2012**, *24*, 15–24. [CrossRef]
54. Thomas, V.; Halloran, B.A.; Ambalavanan, N.; Catledge, S.A.; Vohra, Y.K. In vitro studies on the effect of particle size on macrophage responses to nanodiamond wear debris. *Acta Biomater.* **2012**, *8*, 1939–1947. [CrossRef] [PubMed]
55. Puzyr, A.; Neshumayev, D.; Tarskikh, S.; Makarskaya, G.; Dolmatov, V.; Bondar, V. Destruction of human blood cells in interaction with detonation nanodiamonds in experiments in vitro. *Diam. Relat. Mater.* **2004**, *13*, 2020–2023. [CrossRef]
56. Dworak, N.; Wnuk, M.; Zebrowski, J.; Bartosz, G.; Lewinska, A. Genotoxic and mutagenic activity of diamond nanoparticles in human peripheral lymphocytes in vitro. *Carbon* **2014**, *68*, 763–776. [CrossRef]
57. Solarska, K.; Gajewska, A.; Kaczorowski, W.; Bartosz, G.; Mitura, K. Effect of nanodiamond powders on the viability and production of reactive oxygen and nitrogen species by human endothelial cells. *Diam. Relat. Mater.* **2012**, *21*, 107–113. [CrossRef]

58. Marcon, L.; Riquet, F.; Vicogne, D.; Szunerits, S.; Bodart, J.-F.; Boukherroub, R. Cellular and in vivo toxicity of functionalized nanodiamond in Xenopus embryos. *J. Mater. Chem.* **2010**, *20*, 8064–8069. [CrossRef]
59. Stone, V.; Shaw, J.; Brown, D.; MacNee, W.; Faux, S.; Donaldson, K. The role of oxidative stress in the prolonged inhibitory effect of ultrafine carbon black on epithelial cell function. *Toxicol. Vitr.* **1998**, *12*, 649–659. [CrossRef]
60. Vesterdal, L.K.; Danielsen, P.H.; Folkmann, J.K.; Jespersen, L.F.; Aguilar-Pelaez, K.; Roursgaard, M.; Loft, S.; Møller, P. Accumulation of lipids and oxidatively damaged DNA in hepatocytes exposed to particles. *Toxicol. Appl. Pharmacol.* **2014**, *274*, 350–360. [CrossRef]
61. Jacobsen, N.R.; Saber, A.T.; White, P.; Møller, P.; Pojana, G.; Vogel, U.; Loft, S.; Gingerich, J.; Soper, L.; Douglas, G.R.; et al. Increased mutant frequency by carbon black, but not quartz, in thelacZ andcII transgenes of muta™ mouse lung epithelial cells. *Environ. Mol. Mutagen.* **2007**, *48*, 451–461. [CrossRef] [PubMed]
62. Tamaoki, J.; Isono, K.; Takeyama, K.; Tagaya, E.; Nakata, J.; Nagai, A. Ultrafine carbon black particles stimulate proliferation of human airway epithelium via EGF receptor-mediated signaling pathway. *Am. J. Physiol. Cell. Mol. Physiol.* **2004**, *287*, L1127–L1133. [CrossRef] [PubMed]
63. Di Giorgio, M.L.; Di Bucchianico, S.; Ragnelli, A.M.; Aimola, P.; Santucci, S.; Poma, A. Effects of single and multi walled carbon nanotubes on macrophages: Cyto and genotoxicity and electron microscopy. *Mutat. Res. Toxicol. Environ. Mutagen.* **2011**, *722*, 20–31. [CrossRef] [PubMed]
64. Mroz, R.M.; Schins, R.P.F.; Li, H.; Drost, E.M.; MacNee, W.; Donaldson, K. Nanoparticle carbon black driven DNA damage induces growth arrest and AP-1 and NFkappaB DNA binding in lung epithelial A549 cell line. *J. Physiol. Pharmacol.* **2007**, *58*, 467–470.
65. Cao, Y.; Roursgaard, M.; Danielsen, P.H.; Møller, P.; Loft, S. Carbon Black Nanoparticles Promote Endothelial Activation and Lipid Accumulation in Macrophages Independently of Intracellular ROS Production. *PLoS ONE* **2014**, *9*, e106711. [CrossRef] [PubMed]
66. Jacobsen, N.R.; Pojana, G.; White, P.; Møller, P.; Cohn, C.A.; Korsholm, K.S.; Vogel, U.; Marcomini, A.; Loft, S.; Wallin, H. Genotoxicity, cytotoxicity, and reactive oxygen species induced by single-walled carbon nanotubes and C_{60} fullerenes in the FE1-Muta™Mouse lung epithelial cells. *Environ. Mol. Mutagen.* **2008**, *49*, 476–487. [CrossRef]
67. Totsuka, Y.; Higuchi, T.; Imai, T.; Nishikawa, A.; Nohmi, T.; Kato, T.; Masuda, S.; Kinae, N.; Hiyoshi, K.; Ogo, S.; et al. Genotoxicity of nano/microparticles in in vitro micronuclei, in vivo comet and mutation assay systems. *Part. Fibre Toxicol.* **2009**, *6*, 23. [CrossRef]
68. Dhawan, A.; Taurozzi, J.S.; Pandey, A.K.; Shan, W.; Miller, S.M.; Hashsham, S.A.; Tarabara, V.V. Stable Colloidal Dispersions of C_{60} Fullerenes in Water: Evidence for Genotoxicity†. *Environ. Sci. Technol.* **2006**, *40*, 7394–7401. [CrossRef]
69. Yamawaki, H.; Iwai, N. Cytotoxicity of water-soluble fullerene in vascular endothelial cells. *Am. J. Physiol. Physiol.* **2006**, *290*, C1495–C1502. [CrossRef]
70. Cui, D.; Tian, F.; Ozkan, C.S.; Wang, M.; Gao, H. Effect of single wall carbon nanotubes on human HEK293 cells. *Toxicol. Lett.* **2005**, *155*, 73–85. [CrossRef]
71. Wick, P.; Manser, P.; Limbach, L.K.; Dettlaff-Weglikowska, U.; Krumeich, F.; Roth, S.; Stark, W.J.; Bruinink, A. The degree and kind of agglomeration affect carbon nanotube cytotoxicity. *Toxicol. Lett.* **2007**, *168*, 121–131. [CrossRef] [PubMed]
72. Jia, G.; Wang, H.; Yan, L.; Wang, X.; Pei, R.; Yan, T.; Zhao, Y.; Guo, X. Cytotoxicity of Carbon Nanomaterials: Single-Wall Nanotube, Multi-Wall Nanotube, and Fullerene. *Environ. Sci. Technol.* **2005**, *39*, 1378–1383. [CrossRef]
73. Pantarotto, D.; Briand, J.P.; Prato, M.; Bianco, A. Translocation of bioactive peptides across cell membranes by carbon nanotubes. *Chem. Commun.* **2004**, 16–17. [CrossRef] [PubMed]
74. Shvedova, A.; Castranova, V.; Kisin, E.; Schwegler-Berry, D.; Murray, A.; Gandelsman, V.; Maynard, A.; Baron, P. Exposure to Carbon Nanotube Material: Assessment of Nanotube Cytotoxicity using Human Keratinocyte Cells. *J. Toxicol. Environ. Health Part A* **2003**, *66*, 1909–1926. [CrossRef] [PubMed]
75. Francis, A.P.; Devasena, T. Toxicity of carbon nanotubes: A review. *Toxicol. Ind. Health* **2018**, *34*, 200–210. [CrossRef] [PubMed]
76. Sayes, C.M.; Liang, F.; Hudson, J.L.; Mendez, J.; Guo, W.; Beach, J.M.; Moore, V.C.; Doyle, C.D.; West, J.L.; Billups, W.E.; et al. Functionalization density dependence of single-walled carbon nanotubes cytotoxicity in vitro. *Toxicol. Lett.* **2006**, *161*, 135–142. [CrossRef] [PubMed]

77. Pacurari, M.; Yin, X.J.; Zhao, J.; Ding, M.; Leonard, S.S.; Schwegler-Berry, D.; Ducatman, B.S.; Sbarra, D.; Hoover, M.D.; Castranova, V.; et al. Raw Single-Wall Carbon Nanotubes Induce Oxidative Stress and Activate MAPKs, AP-1, NF-κB, and Akt in Normal and Malignant Human Mesothelial Cells. *Environ. Health Perspect.* **2008**, *116*, 1211–1217. [CrossRef]
78. Kisin, E.R.; Murray, A.R.; Keane, M.J.; Shi, X.-C.; Schwegler-Berry, D.; Gorelik, O.; Arepalli, S.; Castranova, V.; Wallace, W.E.; Kagan, V.E.; et al. Single-walled Carbon Nanotubes: Geno- and Cytotoxic Effects in Lung Fibroblast V79 Cells. *J. Toxicol. Environ. Health Part A* **2007**, *70*, 2071–2079.
79. Hirano, S.; Kanno, S.; Furuyama, A. Multi-walled carbon nanotubes injure the plasma membrane of macrophages. *Toxicol. Appl. Pharmacol.* **2008**, *232*, 244–251. [CrossRef]
80. Monteiro-Riviere, N.A.; Nemanich, R.J.; Inman, A.O.; Wang, Y.Y.; Riviere, J.E. Multi-walled carbon nanotube interactions with human epidermal keratinocytes. *Toxicol. Lett.* **2005**, *155*, 377–384. [CrossRef]
81. Ding, L.; Stilwell, J.; Zhang, T.; Elboudwarej, O.; Jiang, H.; Selegue, J.P.; Cooke, P.A.; Gray, J.W.; Chen, F.F. Molecular Characterization of the Cytotoxic Mechanism of Multiwall Carbon Nanotubes and Nano-Onions on Human Skin Fibroblast. *Nano Lett.* **2005**, *5*, 2448–2464. [CrossRef] [PubMed]
82. Bottini, M.; Bruckner, S.; Nika, K.; Bottini, N.; Bellucci, S.; Magrini, A.; Bergamaschi, A.; Mustelin, T. Multi-walled carbon nanotubes induce T lymphocyte apoptosis. *Toxicol. Lett.* **2006**, *160*, 121–126. [CrossRef] [PubMed]
83. Yao, K.; Lv, X.; Zheng, G.; Chen, Z.; Jiang, Y.; Zhu, X.; Wang, Z.; Cai, Z. Effects of Carbon Quantum Dots on Aquatic Environments: Comparison of Toxicity to Organisms at Different Trophic Levels. *Environ. Sci. Technol.* **2018**, *52*, 14445–14451. [CrossRef] [PubMed]
84. Zheng, X.; Shao, D.; Li, J.; Song, Y.; Chen, Y.; Pan, Y.; Zhu, S.; Yang, B.; Chen, L. Single and repeated dose toxicity of citric acid-based carbon dots and a derivative in mice. *RSC Adv.* **2015**, *5*, 91398–91406. [CrossRef]
85. Jiang, D.; Chen, Y.; Li, N.; Li, W.; Wang, Z.; Zhu, J.; Zhang, H.; Liu, B.; Xu, S. Synthesis of Luminescent Graphene Quantum Dots with High Quantum Yield and Their Toxicity Study. *PLoS ONE* **2015**, *10*, e0144906. [CrossRef] [PubMed]
86. Wang, Z.G.; Zhou, R.; Jiang, D.; Song, J.E.; Xu, Q.; Si, J.; Chen, Y.P.; Zhou, X.; Gan, L.; Li, J.Z.; et al. Toxicity of Graphene Quantum Dots in Zebrafish Embryo. *Biomed. Environ. Sci.* **2015**, *28*, 341–351. [PubMed]
87. Chong, Y.; Ma, Y.; Shen, H.; Tu, X.; Zhou, X.; Xu, J.; Dai, J.; Fan, S.; Zhang, Z. The in vitro and in vivo toxicity of graphene quantum dots. *Biomaterials* **2014**, *35*, 5041–5048. [CrossRef] [PubMed]
88. Nurunnabi, M.; Khatun, Z.; Huh, K.M.; Park, S.Y.; Lee, D.Y.; Cho, K.J.; Lee, Y.K. In Vivo Biodistribution and Toxicology of Carboxylated Graphene Quantum Dots. *ACS Nano* **2013**, *7*, 6858–6867. [CrossRef] [PubMed]
89. Mohan, N.; Chen, C.S.; Hsieh, H.H.; Wu, Y.C.; Chang, H.C. In Vivo Imaging and Toxicity Assessments of Fluorescent Nanodiamonds in Caenorhabditis elegans. *Nano Lett.* **2010**, *10*, 3692–3699. [CrossRef]
90. Yuan, Y.; Wang, X.; Jia, G.; Liu, J.H.; Wang, T.; Gu, Y.; Yang, S.T.; Zhen, S.; Wang, H.; Liu, Y. Pulmonary toxicity and translocation of nanodiamonds in mice. *Diam. Relat. Mater.* **2010**, *19*, 291–299. [CrossRef]
91. Kamata, H.; Tasaka, S.; Inoue, K.I.; Miyamoto, K.; Nakano, Y.; Shinoda, H.; Kimizuka, Y.; Fujiwara, H.; Ishii, M.; Hasegawa, N.; et al. Carbon black nanoparticles enhance bleomycin-induced lung inflammatory and fibrotic changes in mice. *Exp. Biol. Med.* **2011**, *236*, 315–324. [CrossRef] [PubMed]
92. Inoue, K.-I.; Yanagisawa, R.; Koike, E.; Nakamura, R.; Ichinose, T.; Tasaka, S.; Kiyono, M.; Takano, H. Effects of Carbon Black Nanoparticles on Elastase-Induced Emphysematous Lung Injury in Mice. *Basic Clin. Pharmacol. Toxicol.* **2011**, *108*, 234–240. [CrossRef] [PubMed]
93. Saputra, D.; Yoon, J.H.; Park, H.; Heo, Y.; Yang, H.; Lee, E.J.; Lee, S.; Song, C.W.; Lee, K. Inhalation of Carbon Black Nanoparticles Aggravates Pulmonary Inflammation in Mice. *Toxicol. Res.* **2014**, *30*, 83–90. [CrossRef] [PubMed]
94. Lindner, K.; Ströbele, M.; Schlick, S.; Webering, S.; Jenckel, A.; Kopf, J.; Danov, O.; Sewald, K.; Buj, C.; Creutzenberg, O.; et al. Biological effects of carbon black nanoparticles are changed by surface coating with polycyclic aromatic hydrocarbons. *Part. Fibre Toxicol.* **2017**, *14*, 8. [CrossRef] [PubMed]
95. Morimoto, Y.; Hirohashi, M.; Ogami, A.; Oyabu, T.; Myojo, T.; Nishi, K.-I.; Kadoya, C.; Todoroki, M.; Yamamoto, M.; Murakami, M.; et al. Inflammogenic effect of well-characterized fullerenes in inhalation and intratracheal instillation studies. *Part. Fibre Toxicol.* **2010**, *7*, 4. [CrossRef] [PubMed]

96. Fujita, K.; Morimoto, Y.; Ogami, A.; Myojyo, T.; Tanaka, I.; Shimada, M.; Wang, W.-N.; Endoh, S.; Uchida, K.; Nakazato, T.; et al. Gene expression profiles in rat lung after inhalation exposure to C_{60} fullerene particles. *Toxicology* **2009**, *258*, 47–55. [CrossRef] [PubMed]
97. Park, E.J.; Kim, H.; Kim, Y.; Yi, J.; Choi, K.; Park, K. Carbon fullerenes (C_{60}s) can induce inflammatory responses in the lung of mice. *Toxicol. Appl. Pharmacol.* **2010**, *244*, 226–233. [CrossRef] [PubMed]
98. Folkmann, J.K.; Risom, L.; Jacobsen, N.R.; Wallin, H.; Loft, S.; Møller, P. Oxidatively damaged DNA in rats exposed by oral gavage to C_{60} fullerenes and single-walled carbon nanotubes. *Environ. Health Perspect.* **2009**, *117*, 703–708. [CrossRef]
99. Roursgaard, M.; Poulsen, S.S.; Kepley, C.L.; Hammer, M.; Nielsen, G.D.; Larsen, S.T. Polyhydroxylated C_{60}Fullerene (Fullerenol) Attenuates Neutrophilic Lung Inflammation in Mice. *Basic Clin. Pharmacol. Toxicol.* **2008**, *103*, 386–388. [CrossRef]
100. Kagan, V.E.; Konduru, N.V.; Feng, W.; Allen, B.L.; Conroy, J.; Volkov, Y.; Vlasova, I.I.; Belikova, N.A.; Yanamala, N.; Kapralov, A.; et al. Carbon nanotubes degraded by neutrophil myeloperoxidase induce less pulmonary inflammation. *Nat. Nanotechnol.* **2010**, *5*, 354–359. [CrossRef]
101. Lin, Z.; Ma, L.; Zhu-Ge, X.; Zhang, H.; Lin, B. A comparative study of lung toxicity in rats induced by three types of nanomaterials. *Nanoscale Res. Lett.* **2013**, *8*, 521. [CrossRef] [PubMed]
102. Saber, A.T.; Lamson, J.S.; Jacobsen, N.R.; Ravn-Haren, G.; Hougaard, K.S.; Nyendi, A.N.; Wahlberg, P.; Madsen, A.M.; Jackson, P.; Wallin, H.; et al. Particle-Induced Pulmonary Acute Phase Response Correlates with Neutrophil Influx Linking Inhaled Particles and Cardiovascular Risk. *PLoS ONE* **2013**, *8*, e69020. [CrossRef] [PubMed]
103. Poland, C.A.; Duffin, R.; Kinloch, I.; Maynard, A.; Wallace, W.A.H.; Seaton, A.; Stone, V.; Brown, S.; MacNee, W.; Donaldson, K. Carbon nanotubes introduced into the abdominal cavity of mice show asbestos-like pathogenicity in a pilot study. *Nat. Nanotechnol.* **2008**, *3*, 423–428. [CrossRef] [PubMed]
104. Morimoto, Y.; Hirohashi, M.; Ogami, A.; Oyabu, T.; Myojo, T.; Todoroki, M.; Yamamoto, M.; Hashiba, M.; Mizuguchi, Y.; Lee, B.W.; et al. Pulmonary toxicity of well-dispersed multi-wall carbon nanotubes following inhalation and intratracheal instillation. *Nanotoxicology* **2012**, *6*, 587–599. [CrossRef] [PubMed]
105. Muller, J.; Huaux, F.; Moreau, N.; Misson, P.; Heilier, J.-F.; Delos, M.; Arras, M.; Fonseca, A.; Nagy, J.B.; Lison, D. Respiratory toxicity of multi-wall carbon nanotubes. *Toxicol. Appl. Pharmacol.* **2005**, *207*, 221–231. [CrossRef] [PubMed]
106. Grubek-Jaworska, H.; Nejman, P.; Czumińska, K.; Przybyłowski, T.; Huczko, A.; Lange, H.; Bystrzejewski, M.; Baranowski, P.; Chazan, R. Preliminary results on the pathogenic effects of intratracheal exposure to one-dimensional nanocarbons. *Carbon* **2006**, *44*, 1057–1063. [CrossRef]
107. Boisen, A.M.Z.; Shipley, T.; Jackson, P.; Wallin, H.; Nellemann, C.; Vogel, U.; Yauk, C.L.; Hougaard, K.S. In utero exposure to nanosized carbon black (Printex90) does not induce tandem repeat mutations in female murine germ cells. *Reprod. Toxicol.* **2013**, *41*, 45–48. [CrossRef] [PubMed]
108. Driscoll, K.E.; Carter, J.M.; Howard, B.W.; Hassenbein, D.G.; Pepelko, W.; Baggs, R.B.; Oberdörster, G. Pulmonary Inflammatory, Chemokine, and Mutagenic Responses in Rats after Subchronic Inhalation of Carbon Black. *Toxicol. Appl. Pharmacol.* **1996**, *136*, 372–380. [CrossRef] [PubMed]
109. Rittinghausen, S.; Bellmann, B.; Creutzenberg, O.; Ernst, H.; Kolling, A.; Mangelsdorf, I.; Kellner, R.; Beneke, S.; Ziemann, C. Evaluation of immunohistochemical markers to detect the genotoxic mode of action of fine and ultrafine dusts in rat lungs. *Toxicology* **2013**, *303*, 177–186. [CrossRef]
110. Kyjovska, Z.O.; Jacobsen, N.R.; Saber, A.T.; Bengtson, S.; Jackson, P.; Wallin, H.; Vogel, U. DNA damage following pulmonary exposure by instillation to low doses of carbon black (Printex 90) nanoparticles in mice. *Environ. Mol. Mutagen.* **2015**, *56*, 41–49. [CrossRef]
111. Bourdon, J.A.; Saber, A.T.; Halappanavar, S.; Jackson, P.A.; Wu, D.; Hougaard, K.S.; Jacobsen, N.R.; Williams, A.; Vogel, U.; Wallin, H.; et al. Carbon black nanoparticle intratracheal installation results in large and sustained changes in the expression of miR-135b in mouse lung. *Environ. Mol. Mutagen.* **2012**, *53*, 462–468. [CrossRef] [PubMed]
112. Li, Z.; Hulderman, T.; Salmen, R.; Chapman, R.; Leonard, S.S.; Young, S.H.; Shvedova, A.; Luster, M.I.; Simeonova, P.P. Cardiovascular effects of pulmonary exposure to single-wall carbon nanotubes. *Environ. Health Perspect.* **2007**, *115*, 377–382. [CrossRef] [PubMed]

113. Takagi, A.; Hirose, A.; Nishimura, T.; Fukumori, N.; Ogata, A.; Ohashi, N.; Kitajima, S.; Kanno, J. Induction of mesothelioma in p53+/− mouse by intraperitoneal application of multi-wall carbon nanotube. *J. Toxicol. Sci.* **2008**, *33*, 105–116. [CrossRef] [PubMed]
114. Yamaguchi, A.; Fujitani, T.; Ohyama, K.I.; Nakae, D.; Hirose, A.; Nishimura, T.; Ogata, A. Effects of sustained stimulation with multi-wall carbon nanotubes on immune and inflammatory responses in mice. *J. Toxicol. Sci.* **2012**, *37*, 177–189. [CrossRef] [PubMed]

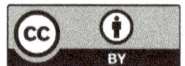

© 2019 by the authors. Licensee MDPI, Basel, Switzerland. This article is an open access article distributed under the terms and conditions of the Creative Commons Attribution (CC BY) license (http://creativecommons.org/licenses/by/4.0/).

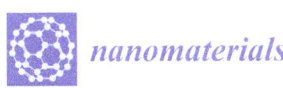

Article

Effect of Surface Coating of Gold Nanoparticles on Cytotoxicity and Cell Cycle Progression

Qian Li, Chun Huang, Liwei Liu, Rui Hu * and Junle Qu

Key Laboratory of Optoelectronic Devices and Systems of Ministry of Education and Guangdong Province, College of Optoelectronic Engineering, Shenzhen University, Shenzhen 518060, China; liqian123@szu.edu.cn (Q.L.); huangchun1190@163.com (C.H.); liulw@szu.edu.cn (L.L.); jlqu@szu.edu.cn (J.Q.)
* Correspondence: rhu@szu.edu.cn; Tel.: +86-0755-2673-3319; Fax: +86-0755-2653-6237

Received: 26 November 2018; Accepted: 12 December 2018; Published: 17 December 2018

Abstract: Gold nanoparticles (GNPs) are usually wrapped with biocompatible polymers in biomedical field, however, the effect of biocompatible polymers of gold nanoparticles on cellular responses are still not fully understood. In this study, GNPs with/without polymer wrapping were used as model probes for the investigation of cytotoxicity and cell cycle progression. Our results show that the bovine serum albumin (BSA) coated GNPs (BSA-GNPs) had been transported into lysosomes after endocytosis. The lysosomal accumulation had then led to increased binding between kinesin 5 and microtubules, enhanced microtubule stabilization, and eventually induced G_2/M arrest through the regulation of cadherin 1. In contrast, the bare GNPs experienced lysosomal escape, resulting in microtubule damage and G_0/G_1 arrest through the regulation of proliferating cell nuclear antigen. Overall, our findings showed that both naked and BSA wrapped gold nanoparticles had cytotoxicity, however, they affected cell proliferation via different pathways. This will greatly help us to regulate cell responses for different biomedical applications.

Keywords: cell cycle; nanoparticle location; surface biocompatibility; microtubule; proteomics

1. Introduction

As the engineering of nanoparticles has been extensively developed over the past decades, various nanoparticles with unique physical and chemical properties have been designed for potential medical applications [1,2]. Improving our understanding of the interactions between nanoparticles and biological systems, especially at the cellular level, is crucial for their risk control and for evaluating their potential applications as drug delivery vehicles or therapeutic agents [3]. The study of interactions between nanoparticles and biological systems, with an emphasis on elucidating the relationship between the physicochemical properties of nanoparticles and biological responses, is essential [4,5]. Such studies are important prerequisites for designing and engineering nanoparticles with intentionally enhanced or suppressed cellular responses and toxicity. However, the mechanisms mediating cellular responses to nanoparticles remain unclear, particularly about the effects of nanoparticles on cell cycle arrest at different phases.

As the cell cycle is closely related to cell proliferation and cytotoxicity, elucidating the mechanisms of different nanostructures on the regulation of cell cycle will be of great importance [6]. Nanoparticles have been shown to cause cell cycle arrest, including G_2/M and G_0/G_1 arrest. The type and extent of cell cycle arrest varies depending on the composition, size, size distribution, surface modification, and subsequent surface derivatization of nanoparticles [7–9]. G_0/G_1 arrest can be caused by DNA damage and microtubule damage, while nanoparticles in combination with oxidative stress and/or lysosome rupture could lead to G_0/G_1 arrest. However, the mechanisms and the factors behind the G_2/M cell cycle arrest caused by nanoparticles are still unclear. Recently, Mahmoudi et al. speculated that the effects of nanoparticles on the cell cycle may depend on the intracellular location of the nanoparticles [6]. Additionally, Choudhury et al. reported that gold nanoparticles (GNPs) with lysosomal escape ability localized to the tubulin/microtubule system and caused cell cycle arrest at G_0/G_1 phase through induction of microtubule damage [10]. However, whether the intracellular localization of nanoparticles is linked with G_2/M cell cycle arrest is still unknown.

GNPs have been recognized as promising nanoprobes in biomedical applications for clinical translation. Although they were once believed to be biocompatible, they are now known to cause cell cycle arrest and show unexpected toxicity to mammalian cells. In addition, the results of various studies have differed due to the use of GNPs with different physicochemical properties [10–12]. Thus, further studies are needed to evaluate the mechanisms through which GNPs cause cell cycle arrest. In this study, two types of GNPs with cetyltrimethylammonium bromide (CTAB)/bovine serum albumin (BSA) coatings were evaluated using raw 264.7 macrophage cells. Although there are earlier reports about BSA coated gold nanoparticles, their mechanism for modulating the cell cycle is still unknown. The correlations between biocompatibility, subcellular localization and cell cycle arrest of GNPs were investigated. We believe that our findings will improve the current understanding of the mechanisms behind which nanoparticles induce cell cycle arrest at different phases.

2. Materials and Methods

2.1. Materials

Hydrogen tetrachloroaurate ($HAuCl_4 \cdot 3H_2O$), silver nitrate ($AgNO_3$), CTAB, sodium salicylate, ascorbic acid, sodium citrate, poly(4-styrenesulfonic acid-co-maleic acid) sodium salt (PSSMA), and BSA were obtained from Sigma (Saint Louis, MO, USA). Rat monoclonal anti-α-tubulin antibodies conjugated with Alexa Fluor 647, rat monoclonal anti-α-tubulin antibodies and horseradish peroxidase (HRP)-labeled goat anti-rat IgG were purchased from Abcam (Cambridge, UK). Dulbecco's modified Eagle's medium (DMEM), fetal bovine serum (FBS), and phosphate-buffered saline (PBS) were purchased from Gibco (New York, NY, USA). The annexin V-fluorescein isothiocyanate (FITC) apoptosis detection kit, and propidium iodide (PI) cell cycle assay kit, phalloidin-FITC cytopainter, and 4′,6-diamidino-2-phenylindole (DAPI) were purchased from Beyotime (Shanghai, China). Lyso Tracker Green DND-26 was obtained from Invitrogen (Carlsbad, CA, USA).

2.2. Preparation and Characterization of GNPs

GNPs were prepared as previously described [13]. Briefly, 5 mL of 0.5 mM $HAuCl_4$ was mixed with 5 mL of 0.2 M CTAB solution, and 1 mL of 6 mM $NaBH_4$ was then added. The solution was stirred for 2 min and incubated for 30 min to prepare the seed solution. To prepare colorless growth solution, 9.0 g CTAB plus 0.8 g sodium salicylate were dissolved in 250 mL warm water. Next, 6 mL of 4 mM $AgNO_3$ solution and 1 mL of 0.064 M ascorbic acid were added. Finally, 0.8 mL seed solution was injected into the growth solution, stirred for 30 s and left undisturbed at 30 °C for 12 h for GNP growth. To obtain CTAB-GNPs, the precipitates after centrifugation were re-dispersed in 10 mL distilled water. According to previous reports [14,15], the CTAB-GNPs were further coated with the polyelectrolyte PSSMA and BSA under stirring to obtain BSA-GNPs.

The morphology of the nanoparticles was observed by TEM at an accelerating voltage of 100 kV (JEOL Co., Tokyo, Japan). The size stability of nanoparticles was determined with a Brooke Haven Nanosizer at 37 °C with GNPs in DMEM medium (pH 7.4) at the concentration of 15 pM. Ultraviolet-visible (UV-vis) measurements were carried out using a Shimadzu UV 2700 spectrophotometer (Kyoto, Japan).

2.3. Flow Cytometry Analysis of the Cell Cycle and Apoptosis

RAW264.7 cells were obtained from the Shanghai Institutes for Biological Sciences (Shanghai, China) and routinely cultured in DMEM supplemented with 10% FBS at 37 °C in a humidified atmosphere with 5% CO_2 in air. Progression of cells through the cell cycle was examined by flow cytometry in RAW264.7 cells treated with GNPs. RAW264.7 cells were plated at 4×10^4 cells/cm^2 in six-well plates and grown for 18 h. After incubation of cells with GNPs (0–30 pM) for 2 h, the medium was replaced with DMEM, and the cells were incubated for an additional 0–14 h. The interaction time between cells and GNPs in this study refers to incubation with GNPs in DMEM for 2 h plus incubation with GNP-free DMEM for 0–14 h. The cells were fixed in 70% ethanol, and DNA was stained with PI in the presence of 40 mg/mL DNase-free RNase A for 30 min at 37 °C in the dark. Cell cycle analysis was performed using flow cytometry according to the manufacturer's instructions. Early apoptotic cells were quantified by annexin V-FITC, whereas late apoptotic and necrotic cells were identified by PI staining. After treatment with GNPs, cells were trypsinized, harvested, washed with PBS, incubated with annexin V-FITC/PI for 15 min at room temperature in the dark, and analyzed on a flow cytometer (FACSCalibur BD, CA, USA).

2.4. Confocal Microscopy Analysis

Intracellular localization of GNPs was visualized using a Leica SP8 fluorescence confocal microscope (Wetzlar, Germany). RAW264.7 cells were treated with GNPs as described in the previous section and then co-incubated with Lyso Tracker Green DND-26 at 37 °C for 0.5 h. After washing with PBS, live cell imaging of green fluorescence with Lyso Tracker Green and diffusion reflection of GNPs irradiated at 630 nm were measured using a Leica SP8 (Wetzlar, Germany).

The morphology of the cytoskeleton was determined by immuno-staining RAW264.7 cells with a microtubule/microfilament fluorescent probe. Briefly, cells were fixed with 4% formaldehyde for 10 min, permeabilized with 0.1% Triton X-100 for 5 min, blocked with 1% BSA for 1 h, and then incubated with anti-tubulin antibodies conjugated with Alexa Fluor 647 and/or phalloidin-FITC according to the manufacturer's instructions for staining microfilament and microtubules. The cells were co-incubated with DAPI for nuclear staining. Polychromatic images of cells were measured using a Leica SP8 for green fluorescence indicating microfilament, red fluorescence indicating microtubules, and blue fluorescence indicating nuclei. Diffusion reflection of GNPs was defined as yellow, green, or red to avoid confusion with fluorescence.

2.5. Western Blot Analysis

Changes in the ratios of free tubulin within the polymerized microtubules were measured by western blotting. After treatment with GNPs, cells were lysed with 0.2 mL lysis buffer (20 mM Tris-HCl (pH 6.8), 0.5% NP-40, 1 mM $MgCl_2$, 2 mM EGTA, 1 mM orthovanadate, and 20 mg/mL aprotinin, leupeptin, and pepstatin). Centrifugation yielded soluble tubulin dimers in the supernatant and polymerized microtubules in the pellet. Pellets were solubilized with sodium dodecyl sulfate (SDS) lysis buffer (Beyotime; Shanghai, China). Cell lysates containing equal amounts of protein were separated by SDS-polyacrylamide gel electrophoresis, transferred, probed with specific antibodies against α-tubulin, and detected on X-ray films using the chemiluminescence technique.

2.6. qRT-PCR

RAW264.7 cells were incubated with GNPs and then harvested for examination of gene expression by qRT-PCR. Briefly, total RNA was extracted with TRIzol reagent (CW0580S; CWBIO, Beijing, China). cDNA was then synthesized using a SuperScriptFirst-Strand Synthesis kit (CW2569M; CWBIO). The specific primers used in this study were as follows: *p53*, (forward) 5′-GCTCCTCCCCAGCATCTTA-3′ and (reverse) 5′-GGGCAGTTCAGGGCAAA-3′; kinesin 5A, (forward) 5′-GGCGGAGACTAACAACGAA-3′ and (reverse) 5′-CTTGGAAAATGGGGATGAA-3′; glyceraldehyde 3-phosphate dehydrogenase, (forward) 5′-AAGAAGGTGGTGAAGCAGG-3′ and (reverse) 5′-GAAGGTGGAAGAGTGGGAGT-3′. The relative expression of mRNA was calculated by the $2^{-\Delta\Delta Ct}$ method.

2.7. Proteomics Analysis

Cells were incubated with GNPs (30 pM) for 6 h, and cellular protein was extracted, digested, and desalted. The resulting peptide mixture was labeled with an iTRAQ Reagent-8 plex Multiplex Kit (AB Sciex U.K. Limited, Sheffield, U.K.) according to the manufacturer's instructions. Next, the labeled samples were fractionated using high-performance liquid chromatography (Thermo DINOEX Ultimate 3000 BioRS, Waltham, USA) using a Durashell C18 column (5 μm, 100 Å, 4.6 × 250 mm, Tianjin, China). Liquid chromatography electrospray ionization tandem mass spectrometry (MS/MS) analysis was performed on an AB SCIEX nanoLC-MS/MS (Triple TOF 5600 plus) system. Briefly, samples were chromategraphed on a C18 column (3 μm, 75 μm × 150 mm) with a 90-min gradient elution. Buffer A (0.1% formic acid and 5% acetonitrile) and buffer B (0.1% formic acid and 95% acetonitrile) served as the mobile phase. MS1 spectra were collected in the range of m/z 350–1500 for 250 ms, and the 30 most intense precursor ions were selected for fragmentation. MS2 spectra were collected in the range of m/z 100–1500 for 50 ms. Precursor ions were excluded from reselection for 15 s. The original MS/MS file data were submitted to ProteinPilot Software v4.5 (AB Sciex Pte Ltd. Waltham, MA, USA; https://sciex.com/products/software/proteinpilot-software) for data analysis. For protein identification, Paragon algorithm2, which was integrated into ProteinPilot, was employed against Uniprot Mus musculus 20171124.fasta (84434 items, updated in November 2017) for database searching. The parameters were set as follows: Instrument, TripleTOF 5600; iTRAQ quantification; cysteine modified with iodoacetamide. The biological modifications included ID focus and trypsin digestion, and the quantitate, bias correction, and background correction was used for protein quantification and normalization. Only proteins with at least one unique peptide and an unused value of more than 1.3 were considered for further analysis.

3. Results

3.1. Proertiesof GNPs withBSA/CTABCapping Agents

As the surfactants have poor biocompatibility, several shells such as carbon shells and biopolymer shells have been used to reduce toxicity of surfactants [16]. We chose BSA as a model molecule for its biocompatibility. Zeta potential of CTAB-GNPs and BSA-GNPs are 28.4 ± 2.6 mV and −20.5 ± 2.1 mV respectively, indicating positive CTAB and negative BSA on the surface of GNPs. The physicochemical properties of BSA-GNPs and CTAB-GNPs are shown in Figure 1. Transmission electron microscopy (TEM) showed that both types of nanoparticles were rod shaped with similar particle sizes in distilled water (Figure 1A,B). Although the hydrodynamic diameter deduced from the Stokes-Einstein equation was not accurate when regarding nano-rods as nano-spheres, the diffusion coefficient determined by dynamic light scattering (DLS) was still accurate. The particle size peak can be a signature for determining the nano-rod aggregation formation [17]. DLS analysis showed that the particle size of CTAB-GNPs increased from 45 to 79 nm as the incubation time increased. In contrast, no significant changes in particle size were observed for BSA-GNPs (Figure 1C). These results indicated coating with BSA enhanced the stability of GNPs, which can be attributed to good dispersity of BSA in high salt solution.The extinction spectra of the nanoparticles showed a peak at around 630 nm, which corresponded to the longitudinal surface plasmon resonance of the rod-shaped GNPs (Figure 1D).

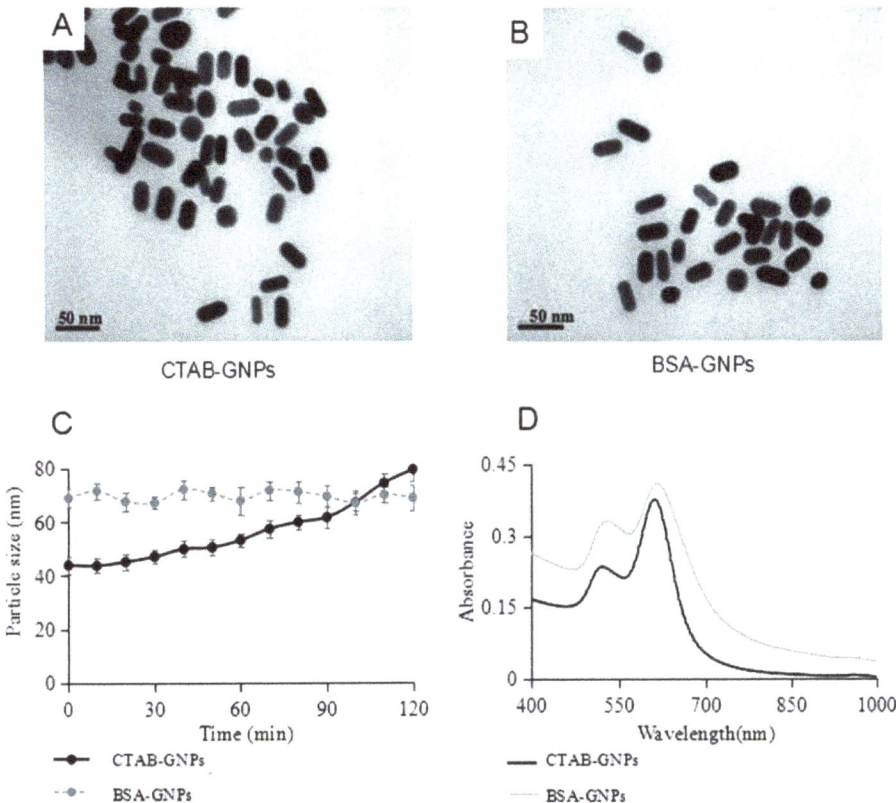

Figure 1. Characterization of GNPs. (**A**) TEM image of CTAB-GNPs in distilled water. (**B**) TEM image of BSA-GNPs in distilled water. (**C**) Hydrodynamic size of GNPs in DMEM. (**D**) UV-vis spectra of GNPs in distilled water.

3.2. Effects of GNPs on the Cell Cycle and Apoptosis

Murine macrophages RAW264.7 were used owing to their strong nanoparticle phagocytosis and short cell cycle period. Apoptosis assays revealed that incubation of RAW264.7 cells with 15 pM of BSA-GNPs yielded 38.82% ± 4.30% early apoptotic cells and 33.98% ± 4.37% late apoptotic cells, whereas incubation of cells with 15 pM of CTAB-GNPs yielded 59.72% ± 1.52% early apoptotic cells and 10.23% ± 1.57% late apoptotic cells (Figure 2A,C). The apoptosis rate increased as the concentration of GNPs increased. Thus, for subsequent cell cycle analyses, we chose a dosage of 15 pM. Compared with the control group (7.71% ± 1.64% in G_2/M phase), 18.54% ± 1.40% of cells were in the G_2/M phase after treatment with 15 pM BSA-GNPs for 2 h. This indicated that BSA-GNPs induced cell cycle arrest at G_2/M phase. Notably, for the cells treated with 15 pM CTAB-GNPs for 2 h, 62.88% ± 3.01% of cells were found to be in the G_0/G_1 phase, compared with 48.56% ± 1.57% in the control group. BSA-GNPs and CTAB-GNPs also induced G_2/M and G_0/G_1 arrest after 16 h of treatment (Figure 2B,D), respectively.

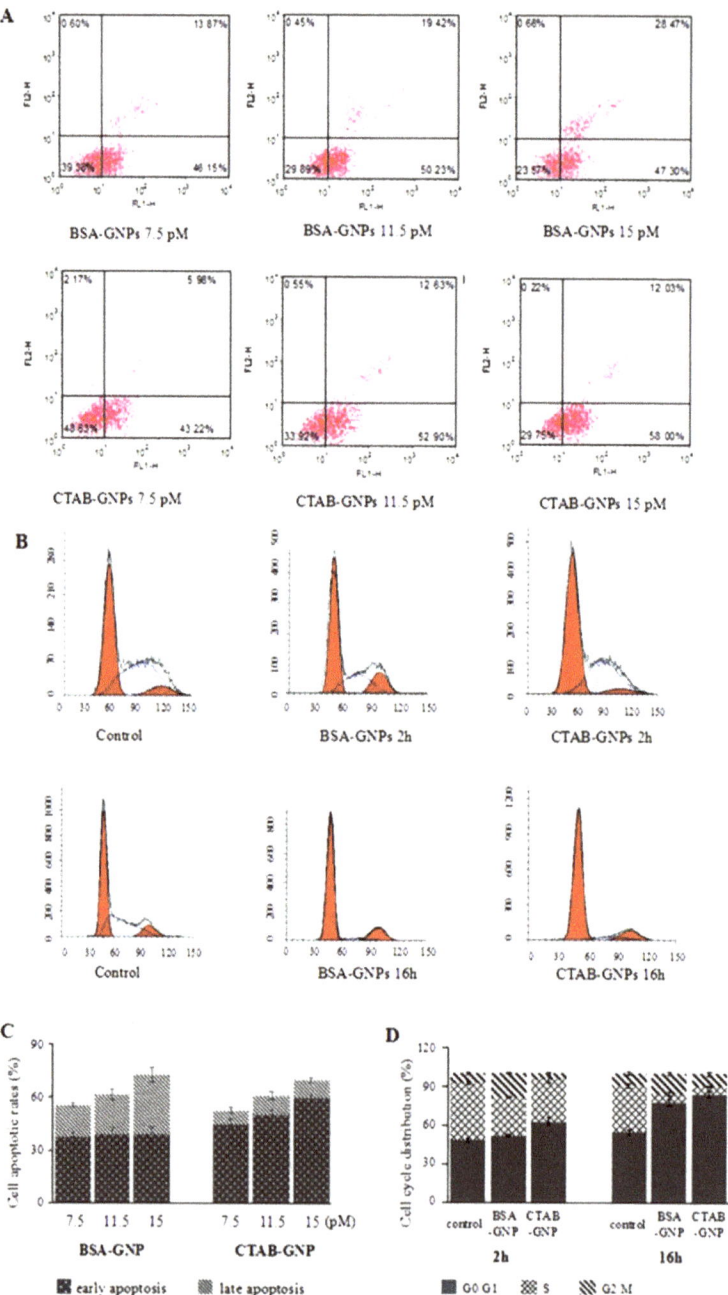

Figure 2. Apoptosis and cell cycle distributions of RAW264.7 cells before and after GNP treatment, with untreated cells used as control. (**A**) Flow cytometry images of GNPs inducing cell apoptosis after incubation for 16 h. (**B**) Flow cytometry images of cell cycle arrest in RAW264.7 cells treated with 15 pM BSA-GNPs and CTAB-GNPs for 2 or 16 h. (**C**) Barchart showing intensity of cell apoptosis. (**D**) Barchart showing distributions of the cell cycle.

3.3. Intracellular Localization of GNPs

Lysosomes, sliding on microtubules, play important roles in the intracellular transportation of nanoparticles [18]. As microtubules greatly affect the cell cycle, interactions of GNPs with lysosomes/microtubules were investigated. Figure 3 shows fluorescent images of GNP-treated cells in which the cell nucleus, lysosomes, microtubules, and GNPs were labeled in different channels. As shown in Figure 3A, the green fluorescence from Lyso Tracker Green DND-26 disappeared in most of the regions of the cells treated with CTAB-GNPs, indicating the disruption of lysosomes by CTAB-GNPs. This could be attributed to the surfactant CTAB, which facilitates lysosome escapees reported in previous reports [19]. However, different results were found in BSA-GNP-treated cells. The colocalization of green fluorescence from lysosomes and scattering reflection from BSA-GNPs (in red) showed that BSA-GNPs were accumulated in lysosomes. In addition, the accumulated green fluorescence of the Lyso Tracker Green DND-26 indicated an accumulation of lysosomes.

Figure 3B,C show the cytoskeleton morphology upon GNP treatment, as determined by laser confocal microscopy. Compared with the PBS treated cells, CTAB-GNPs caused shrinkage of microtubules, microfilaments, and nuclei after 2 h of nanoparticle treatment [20]. Additionally, CTAB-GNPs were aggregated into small circulars with diameters between 0.6–0.9 μm, and they were matched with the red fluorescence from α-tubulin after 16 h of treatment. These suggest that CTAB-GNPs induced tubulin aggregation. In contrast, BSA-GNPs treated cells showed increased microtubule and nuclear organization in the mitosis phase [21]. No overlap between the BSA-GNPs and microtubule-tubulin system was observed after 16 h of nanoparticle treatment.

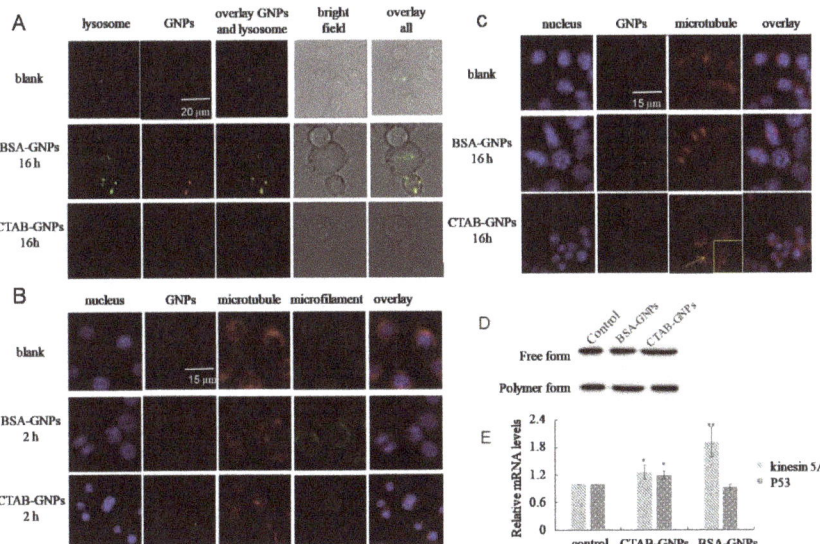

Figure 3. Effect of GNPs on subcellular organelles, with untreated cells used as control. (**A**) Confocal microscopy images of cell lysosome after incubation with GNPs for 16 h, showing colocalization of BSA-GNPs (red) with lysosomes (green). (**B**) Fluorescence microscopy images of cell cytoskeleton after incubation with GNP for 2 h, showing shrinkage of microtubules (red) and microfilaments (green) in CTAB-GNPs and increased microtubules (red) and nuclear (blue) organization in the mitosis phase in BSA-GNPs. (**C**) Fluorescence microscopy images of cell cytoskeleton after incubation with GNP for 16 h, showing colocalization of GNPs (green) with microtubules (red). (**D**) Western blot analysis of free tubulin and polymerized microtubule in cells treated with GNPs. (**E**) Relative mRNA levels of kinesin 5A and P53 in cells treated with GNPs.

3.4. Effects of Nanoparticles On depolymerization/Polymerization of Microtubules

To investigate the potential effects of nanoparticles on the depolymerization/polymerization of microtubules, western blotting was performed after separating the free tubulin from polymerized microtubules. In these cells, treatment with BSA-GNPs increased polymerized microtubules compared with the untreated control cells (Figure 3D), suggesting microtubule stabilization and inhibition of microtubule depolymerization. However, cells treated with CTAB-GNPs showed increased free tubulin, which may be due to the inhibition of microtubule polymerization and assembly of tubulin into small aggregates [10,22].

3.5. Protein Identification and Quantification by Quantitative Real-Time Reverse Transcription Polymerase Chain Reaction (qRT-PCR)

Kinesin 5A is a microtubule motor protein associated with lysosomes and acts as a microtubule polymerase by promoting tubulin polymerization and inhibition of tubulin depolymerization [23,24]. Compared with the control group, the mRNA level of kinesin 5A increased 1.26- and 1.91-fold in CTAB-GNP and BSA-GNP treated cells, respectively (Figure 3E). The increase in kinesin 5A could be attributed to the accumulation of lysosomes on microtubule during GNP transport. However, kinesin 5A levels in CTAB-GNP treated cells were much lower than those in BSA-GNP-treated cells, potentially because of the subsequent lysosome rupture induced by CTAB-GNPs. Overall, the significant increase of kinesin 5A ($p < 0.01$) suggested lysosome accumulation on microtubules and microtubule stabilization in BSA-GNP treated cells. As shown in Figure 3E, p53 mRNA levels were decreased by 8.92% in BSA-GNP-treated cells, yet increased by 1.21fold ($p < 0.05$) in CTAB-GNP treated cells. The increase of P53 can be contributed to microtubule disruption [25].

3.6. Protein Identification and Quantification by Isobaric Tags for Relative and Absolute Quantitation (iTRAQ)

To further explore the cell cycle arrest mechanism induced by GNPs, we used iTRAQ proteomics to identify and quantify protein changes in RAW264.7 cells before and after GNP treatment. In this study, 3341 and 3348distinct proteins were identified using iTRAQ-based proteomic technology in BSA-GNP and CTAB-GNP treatment, respectively (Figure S1a, Supporting Information). To improve our understanding of the roles of these proteins, differentially accumulated protein analysis was based on the fold-change >1.5 or <0.667 ($p < 0.05$). For the cells treated with BSA-GNPs, 159 proteins were found to be differentially expressed compared with the control, including 65 up-regulated and 94 down-regulated proteins. Moreover, 102 proteins were found to be differentially expressed in CTAB-GNP treated cells, including 55 up-regulated and 47 down-regulated proteins. As shown in the Venn diagram, 36 differentially expressed proteins were common in both GNP-treated groups (Figure S1b, Supporting Information). Gene ontology (GO) classification of these differentially expressed proteins were divided into three classes (biological processes, cellular components, and molecular functions). Cells treated with BSA-GNPs or CTAB-GNPs have shown differences in all the three classes (Figure S2, Supporting Information).

3.7. Effects of Nanoparticles on Cell Cycle-Related Protein Expression

Kyoto Encyclopedia of Genes Genomes (KEGG) annotation analysis of all differentially expressed proteins was used to explore the underlying pathways and processes, and the top 10 altered pathways are shown in Figure S3 (Supporting Information). Down-regulation of cell cycle-related proteins was observed following BSA-GNP treatment. Down-regulation of actin cytoskeleton-related proteins, which are closely related to the cell cycle, were observed following CTAB-GNP treatment. We adopted KEGG annotation analysis to explore the underlying pathways of the cell cycle (Figure 4). Our results showed that three of these unique proteins (cadherin 1 (Cdh1), minichromosome maintenance complex component 5 (MCM5), 14-3-3 protein) were related to the cell cycle in BSA-GNP-treated cells. Of these proteins, the expression of Cdh1 increased 2.22 fold in response to mispositioned spindles. Cdh1 is an antagonist of the spindle assembly checkpoint and its over-expression could lead to the silencing of mitotic cyclin-dependent kinase 1 (CDK1) activity and consequently the cell cycle arrest at G_2/M phase. MCM5, which was up-regulated in the transition from the G_0 to G_1/S phase of the cell cycle [26], was decreased 0.59 fold. Therefore, the reduction of MCM5 is implicated in low numbers of cells in the G_0/G_1 and S phases. The 14-3-3 protein zeta/delta, 14-3-3 protein gamma, and 14-3-3 protein tau were down-regulated 0.36–0.57 fold. The 14-3-3 protein directly binds to kinesin heterodimers and acts as a phospho-Ser/Thr-binding factor [27]. Phosphorylation of kinesin 5A inhibits its binding to microtubules [28]. Thus, we conclude that the down-regulation of 14-3-3 has weakened the phosphorylation of kinesin 5A and thus promoted the binding of kinesin 5A to spindle microtubules. As a result, the microtubule was stabilized by BSA-GNPs. In CTAB-GNP treated cells, proliferating cell nuclear antigen (PCNA) protein was up-regulated by 1.52 fold as compared with that in the control group. PCNA, as an accessory factor for DNA polymerases, is up-regulated rapidly in the G_1 phase through early S phase and is then down-regulated in late S and G_2/M phases. Increased levels of PCNA can cause cell cycle arrest in G_0/G_1 through the inactivation of CDK4/6. Moreover, increased levels of p53 and PCNA can contribute to microtubule damage [25,29].

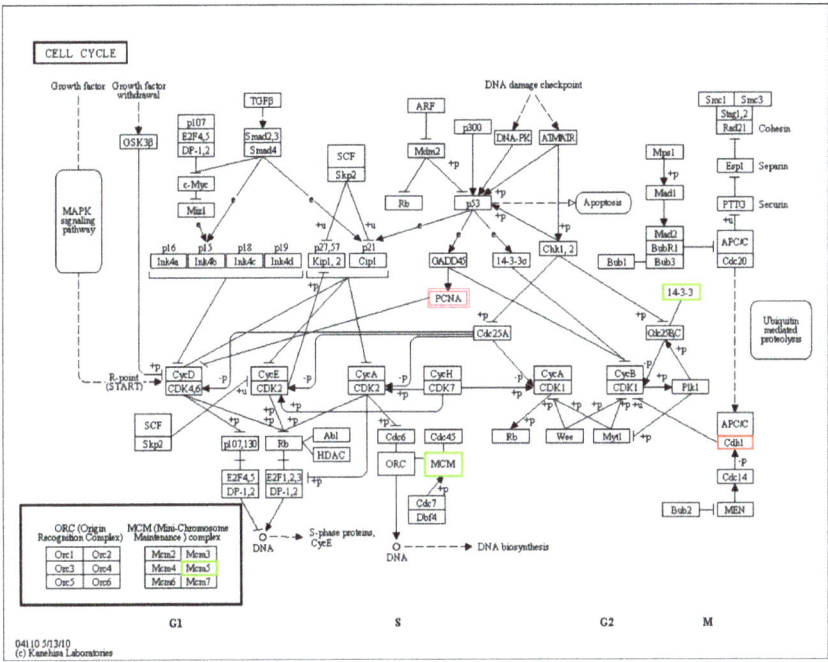

Figure 4. KEGG pathway analysis of the cell cycle in GNP-treated cells. PCNA was up-regulated in CTAB-GNP treated cells. Cdh1 was up-regulated, whereas 14-3-3 protein and MCM5 were down-regulated in BSA-GNP-treated cells. Single line frames refer to BSA-GNPs, and double line frames refer to CTAB-GNPs. Red frames indicate up-regulated proteins, and green frames indicate down-regulated proteins.

4. Discussion

In this study, we found that GNPs causing cell cycle arrest was dependent on biocompatibility of GNP surfaces. Coating of GNPs with biocompatible BSA induced G_2/M arrest through microtubule stabilization, while residual toxic CTAB on the surface of GNPs typically caused cell cycle arrest in G_0/G_1 phase microtubule disruption. Kim et al. have shown that the cell cycle affects the intracellular transport of nanoparticles [30]. Nanoparticles internalized by cells are not exported from cells but are split during G_2/M. Indeed, we found that the intracellular transport/location of nanoparticles had an effect on cell cycle progression (Figure 5). The accumulation of BSA-GNPs in lysosomes increased the level of kinesin 5A and caused subsequent stabilization of microtubules (including the promotion of tubulin polymerization and inhibition of tubulin depolymerization) [23,24], blockage of chromosome segregation, and induction of cell cycle arrest in G_2/M viaCdh1 elevation [31]. In contrast, CTAB on the surface of GNPs caused lysosome/endosome rupture and subsequent microtubule damage through tubulin aggregation and the inhibition of tubulin polymerization. These changes induced G_0/G_1 arrest through the regulation of p53 and PCNA. Overall, biocompatibility properties of GNPs plays an important role in cell cycle progression. Biocompatible coated GNPs could inhibit lysosome rupture caused by residual surfactant and switched G_0/G_1 arrest to G_2/M arrest. Similar results are expected when using other biocompatible molecule coated GNPs, including polyethylene glycol and fluoro-6-deoxy-d-glucose, in accordance with previous reports [32,33].

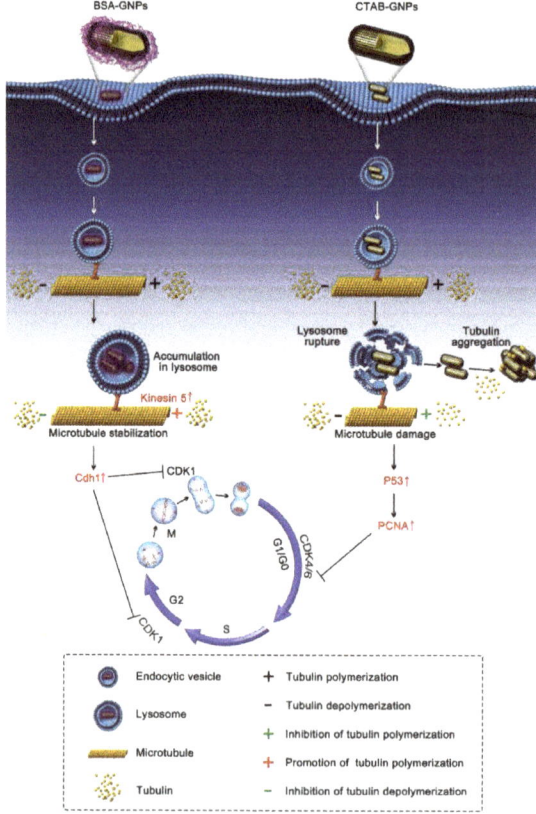

Figure 5. Mechanism through which GNPs causes cell cycle arrest was dependent on the biocompatible property of GNP surface. Coating of GNPs with biocompatible molecules, such as BSA, inhibited lysosome rupture and switched G_0/G_1 arrest to G_2/M arrest. The accumulation of BSA-GNPs in lysosomes increased the level of kinesin 5A and caused subsequent stabilization of microtubules (including promotion of tubulin polymerization and inhibition of tubulin depolymerization), blockage of chromosome segregation, and induction of cell cycle arrest in G_2/M via Cdh1 elevation. In contrast, toxic CTAB on the surface of GNPs caused lysosome rupture and ssubsequent microtubule damage through tubulin aggregation. These changes induced G_0/G_1 arrest through regulation of p53 and PCNA.

Microtubules are the major components of cytoskeletal systems that are responsible for regulation of the cell cycle. Many commonly used drugs, including paclitaxel (a microtubule-stabilizing agent), nocodazole (a microtubule-destabilizing agent), and vinblastine (a microtubule-destabilizing agent) induce G_2/M cell cycle arrest through regulation of microtubules. Choudhury et al. reported that bare GNPs induce G_0/G_1 arrest by causing microtubule damage [10]. In this study, we demonstrated that BSA-coated GNPs stabilized microtubules and caused G_2/M arrest by inducing interactions between lysosomes and microtubules. Nanoparticles are taken up and transported within subcellular structures that are surrounded by one or two layers of membranes, including endosomes, lysosomes, mitochondria, and multivesicular bodies [34]. The motility of these subcellular structures is based on microtubules. Therefore, the transport of nanoparticles can affect dynamic changes in microtubules. Microtubule-interfering drugs affect the cell cycle distribution by impairing the mitotic checkpoint and regulating the activity of cyclins and CDKs. Both stabilization and destabilization of microtubules could impair the mitotic checkpoint and cause G_2/M arrest. For example, microtubule-stabilizing drug paclitaxel regulates the mitotic checkpoint proteins Bub1, CDK1 and CDK2 [35,36]. Microtubule-destabilizing drug nocodazole caused mitotic slippage through precocious activation of Cdh1 and inhibition of CDK1 [37,38]. BSA-GNPs in our study regulated CDK1 through up-regulation of Cdh1, so BSA-GNPs stabilizing microtubules may also lead to a potential cancer therapy.

5. Conclusions

GNPs causing cell cycle arrest was highly dependent on the surface biocompatibility of GNPs. Residual toxic CTAB on the naked GNPs typically caused cell cycle arrest in G_0/G_1 phase, whereas the coating of GNPs with BSA resulted in the inhibition of lysosome rupture ability, microtubule stabilization, and a switch to G_2/M arrest. This will greatly help us to regulate the cell cycle progression through modulating surface coating and biocompatibility of nanoparticles and direct us to set the guidelines for the formulation of nanoparticles in different biomedical applications.More importantly, BSA-GNPs caused G_2/M arrest through microtubule stabilization similarly to the mechanisms of many well-known anticancer drugs, and the recognition of this mechanism could be applied as a new therapeutic target of nanoparticles in tumor therapy.

Supplementary Materials: The following are available online at http://www.mdpi.com/2079-4991/8/12/1063/s1. Additional images related to proteomics analysis of identified and differentially expressed proteins in GNPs treated raw 264.7 cells from iTRAQ proteomics, Gene ontology (GO) classification of differential expressed proteins in GNPs treated cells, Top 10 changed pathways based on proteome analysis in GNPs treated cells.Figure S1: Identified and differentially expressed proteins in GNPs treated raw 264.7 cells from iTRAQ proteomics. Figure S2: Gene ontology (GO) classification of differential expressed proteins. Figure S3: Top 10 changed pathways based on proteome analysis.

Author Contributions: Author Contributions: Q.L. and C.H. conducted the experiments and wrote the paper. L.L. and J.Q. funded the paper. R.H. initiated this study and guided the experiments.

Funding: This research was funded by [National Basic Research Program of China] 2015CB352005; [National Natural Science Foundation of China] 61525503/61620106016/81727804/61722508; [Natural Science Foundation of Guangdong Province Innovation Team] 2014A030312008; and [Science and Technology Innovation Commission of Shenzhen] KQJSCX20170327151457055, JCYJ20170817094609727, JCYJ20170412105003520, JCYJ20150930104948169, JCYJ20160328144746940, GJHZ20160226202139185 and [China Postdoctoral Science Foundation] 2017M622756.

Conflicts of Interest: The authors declare no conflict of interest.

References

1. Wegener, J. Nanoparticles in Biomedical Applications. In *Measuring Biological Impacts of Nanomaterials*; Maximilien, J., Beyazit, S., Rossi, C., Haupt, K., Bui, B.T.S., Eds.; Springer: Cham, Switzerland, 2015; pp. 177–210.
2. Huang, B.; Yan, S.; Xiao, L.; Ji, R.; Yang, L.; Miao, A.J.; Wang, P. Label-free imaging of nanoparticle uptake competition in single cells by hyperspectral stimulated raman scattering. *Small* **2018**, *14*, 1703246. [CrossRef] [PubMed]

3. Wani, M.Y.; Hashim, M.A.; Nabi, F.; Malik, M.A. Nanotoxicity: Dimensional and morphological concerns. *Adv. Phys. Org. Chem.* **2011**, *2011*, 1687–1702. [CrossRef]
4. Nel, A.E.; Mädler, L.; Velegol, D.; Xia, T.; Hoek, E.M.; Somasundaran, P.; Klaessig, F.; Castranova, V.; Thompson, M. Understanding biophysicochemical interactions atthenano-bio interface. *Nat. Mater.* **2009**, *8*, 543–557. [CrossRef]
5. El-Ansary, A.; Al-Daihan, S. On the toxicity of therapeutically used nanoparticles an overview. *J. Toxicol.* **2009**, *2009*, 754810. [CrossRef] [PubMed]
6. Mahmoudi, M.; Azadmanesh, K.; Shokrgozar, M.A.; Journeay, W.; Laurent, S. Effect of nanoparticles on the cell life cycle. *Chem. Rev.* **2011**, *111*, 3407–3432. [CrossRef] [PubMed]
7. Kim, J.A.; Åberg, C.; De Cárcer, G.; Malumbres, M.; Salvati, A.; Dawson, K.A. Correction tolow dose of amino-modified nanoparticles induces cell cycle arrest. *ACS Nano* **2013**, *7*, 7483–7494. [CrossRef] [PubMed]
8. Estevez, H.; Garcia-Lidon, J.C.; Luque-Garcia, J.L.; Camara, C. Effects of chitosan-stabilized selenium nanoparticles on cell proliferation, apoptosis and cell cycle pattern in hepg2 cells: Comparison with other selenospecies. *Colloids Surf. B Biointerfaces* **2014**, *122*, 184–193. [CrossRef]
9. Wu, H.; Zhu, H.; Li, X.; Liu, Z.; Zheng, W.; Chen, T.; Yu, B.; Wong, K.H. Induction of apoptosis and cell cycle arrest in A549 human lung adenocarcinoma cells by surface-capping selenium nanoparticles: An effect enhanced by polysaccharide-protein complexes from Polyporus rhinoceros. *J. Agric. Food Chem.* **2013**, *61*, 9859–9866. [CrossRef]
10. Choudhury, D.; Xavier, P.L.; Chaudhari, K.; John, R.; Dasgupta, A.K.; Pradeep, T.; Chakrabarti, G. Unprecedented inhibition of tubulin polymerization directed by gold nanoparticles inducing cell cycle arrest and apoptosis. *Nanoscale* **2013**, *5*, 4476–4489. [CrossRef]
11. Bergen, J.M.; Von Recum, H.A.; Goodman, T.T.; Massey, A.P.; Pun, S.H. Gold nanoparticles as a versatile platform for optimizing physicochemical parameters for targeted drug delivery. *Macromol. Biosci.* **2006**, *6*, 506–516. [CrossRef]
12. Kumar, C.G.; Poornachandra, Y.; Chandrasekhar, C. Green synthesis of bacterial mediated anti-proliferative gold nanoparticles: Inducing mitotic arrest (G2/M phase) and apoptosis (intrinsic pathway). *Nanoscale* **2015**, *7*, 18738–18750. [CrossRef] [PubMed]
13. Ye, X.; Jin, L.; Caglayan, H.; Chen, J.; Xing, G.; Zheng, C.; Doan-Nguyen, V.; Kang, Y.; Engheta, N.; Kagan, C.R.; et al. Improved size-tunable synthesis of monodisperse gold nanorods through the use of aromatic additives. *ACS Nano* **2012**, *6*, 2804–2817. [CrossRef] [PubMed]
14. Harris, C.M.; Miller, S.G.; Andresen, K.; Thompson, L.B. Quantitative measurement of sodium polystyrene sulfonate adsorption onto CTAB capped gold nanoparticles reveals hard and soft coronas. *J. Colloid Interface Sci.* **2018**, *510*, 39–44. [CrossRef] [PubMed]
15. Talukdar, H.; Kundu, S. Structural and optical behaviour of thin films of protein (BSA)-polyelectrolyte (PAA, PSS) complexes. *AIP Conf. Proc.* **2017**, *1832*, 080011. [CrossRef]
16. Yang, E.; Chou, H.; Tsumura, S.; Nagatsu, M. Surface properties of plasma-functionalized graphite-encapsulated gold nanoparticles prepared by a direct current arc discharge method. *J. Phys. D Appl. Phys.* **2016**, *49*, 185304. [CrossRef]
17. Liu, H.; Nickisha, P.P.; Qun, H. Dynamic light scattering for gold nanorod size characterization and study of nanorod–protein interactions. *Gold Bull.* **2012**, *45*, 187–195. [CrossRef]
18. Liu, M.; Li, Q.; Liang, L.; Li, J.; Wang, K.; Li, J.; Lv, M.; Chen, N.; Song, H.; Lee, J.; et al. Real-time visualization of clustering and intracellular transport of gold nanoparticles by correlative imaging. *Nat. Commun.* **2017**, *8*, 15646. [CrossRef]
19. Liu, S.; Huang, W.; Jin, M.J.; Wang, Q.M.; Zhang, G.L.; Wang, X.M.; Shao, S.; Gao, Z.G. High gene delivery efficiency of alkylated low-molecular-weight polyethylenimine through gemini surfactant-like effect. *Int. J. Nanomed.* **2014**, *9*, 3567–3581. [CrossRef]
20. Gkotzamanidou, M.; Terpos, E.; Munshi, N.C.; Souliotis, V.L.; Dimopoulos, M.A. The state of chromatin condensation, the expression of genes involved in dna damage response and the NDA repair capacity affect the drug sensitivity of pbmcs of myeloma patients treated with melphalan. *Blood* **2015**, *126*, 3628.
21. Lu, D.Y.; Huang, M.; Xu, C.H.; Yang, W.Y.; Hu, C.X.; Lin, L.P.; Tong, L.J.; Li, M.H.; Lu, W.; Zhang, X.W.; et al. Anti-proliferative effects, cell cycle G2/M phase arrest and blocking of chromosome segregation by probimane andMST-16 in human tumor cell lines. *BMC Pharmacol.* **2005**, *5*, 11. [CrossRef]

22. Chen, C.W.; Lee, Y.L.; Liou, J.P.; Liu, Y.H.; Liu, C.W.; Chen, T.Y.; Huang, H.M. A novel tubulin polymerization inhibitor, MPT0B206, down-regulates BCR-ABL expression and induces apoptosis in imatinib-sensitive and imatinib-resistant CML cells. *Apoptosis* **2016**, *21*, 1008–1018. [CrossRef] [PubMed]
23. Cardoso, C.M.; Groth-Pedersen, L.; Høyer-Hansen, M.; Kirkegaard, T.; Corcelle, E.; Andersen, J.S.; Jäättelä, M.; Nylandsted, J. Depletion of kinesin 5B affects lysosomal distribution and stability and induces peri-nuclear accumulation of autophagosomes in cancer cells. *PLoS ONE* **2009**, *4*, 4424. [CrossRef] [PubMed]
24. Chen, Y.; Hancock, W.O. Kinesin-5 is a Microtubule Polymerase. *Nat. Commun.* **2015**, *6*, 8160. [CrossRef] [PubMed]
25. Khan, S.H.; Moritsugu, J.; Wahl, G.M. Differential requirement for p19ARF in the p53-dependent arrest induced by DNA damage, microtubule disruption, and ribonucleotide depletion. *Proc. Natl. Acad. Sci. USA* **2000**, *97*, 3266–3271. [CrossRef] [PubMed]
26. Ohtani, K.; Iwanaga, R.; Nakamura, M.; Ikeda, M.; Yabuta, N.; Tsuruga, H.; Nojima, H. Cell growth-regulated expression of mammalian MCM5 and MCM6 genes mediated by the transcription factor E2F. *Oncogene* **1999**, *18*, 2299–2309. [CrossRef] [PubMed]
27. Ichimura, T.; Wakamiya-Tsuruta, A.; Itagaki, C.; Taoka, M.; Hayano, T.; Natsume, T.; Isobe, T. Phosphorylation-dependent interaction of kinesin light chain 2 and the 14-3-3 protein. *Biochemistry* **2002**, *41*, 5566–5572. [CrossRef]
28. Avunie-Masala, R.; Movshovich, N.; Nissenkorn, Y.; Gerson-Gurwitz, A.; Fridman, V.; Kõivomägi, M.; Loog, M.; Hoyt, M.A.; Zaritsky, A.; Gheber, L. Phospho-regulation of kinesin-5 during anaphase spindle elongation. *J. Cell Sci.* **2011**, *124*, 873–878. [CrossRef]
29. Baschal, E.E.; Chen, K.J.; Elliott, L.G.; Herring, M.J.; Verde, S.C.; Wolkow, T.D. The fission yeast dna structure checkpoint protein Rad26$^{Atrip/Lcd1/Uvsd}$ accumulates in the cytoplasm following microtubule destabilization. *BMC Cell Biol.* **2006**, *7*, 32. [CrossRef]
30. Kim, J.A.; Åberg, C.; Salvati, A.; Dawson, K.A. Role of cell cycle on the cellular uptake and dilution of nanoparticles in a cell population. *Nat. Nanotechnol.* **2011**, *7*, 62–68. [CrossRef]
31. Touati, S.A.; Buffin, E.; Cladière, D.; Hached, K.; Rachez, C.; van Deursen, J.M.; Wassmann, K. Mouse oocytes depend on BubR1 for proper chromosome segregation but not for prophase I arrest. *Nat. Commun.* **2015**, *6*, 6946. [CrossRef]
32. Roa, W.; Zhang, X.; Guo, L.; Shaw, A.; Hu, X.; Xiong, Y.; Gulavita, S.; Patel, S.; Sun, X.; Chen, J.; et al. Gold nanoparticle sensitize radiotherapy of prostate cancer cells by regulation of the cell cycle. *Nanotechnology* **2009**, *20*, 375101. [CrossRef] [PubMed]
33. Uz, M.; Bulmus, V.; Alsoy Altinkaya, S. Effect of PEG grafting density and hydrodynamic volume on gold nanoparticle–cell interactions: An investigation on cell cycle, apoptosis, and DNA damage. *Langmuir* **2016**, *32*, 5997–6009. [CrossRef] [PubMed]
34. Li, Q.; Liu, C.G.; Yu, Y. Separation of monodisperse alginate nanoparticles and effect of particle size on transport of vitamin E. *Carbohydr. Polym.* **2015**, *124*, 274–279. [CrossRef] [PubMed]
35. Sudo, T.; Nitta, M.; Saya, H.; Ueno, N.T. Dependence of paclitaxel sensitivity on a functional spindle assembly checkpoint. *Cancer Res.* **2004**, *64*, 2502–2508. [CrossRef] [PubMed]
36. Nakayama, S.; Torikoshi, Y.; Takahashi, T.; Yoshida, T.; Sudo, T.; Matsushima, T.; Kawasaki, Y.; Katayama, A.; Gohda, K.; Hortobagyi, G.N.; et al. Prediction of paclitaxel sensitivity by CDK1 and CDK2 activity in human breast cancer cells. *Breast Cancer Res.* **2009**, *11*, R12. [CrossRef] [PubMed]
37. Toda, K.; Naito, K.; Mase, S.; Ueno, M.; Uritani, M.; Yamamoto, A.; Ushimaru, T. APC/C-Cdh1-dependent anaphase and telophase progression during mitotic slippage. *Cell Div.* **2012**, *7*, 4. [CrossRef] [PubMed]
38. Chan, Y.W.; Ma, H.T.; Wong, W.; Ho, C.C.; On, K.F.; Poon, R.Y. CDK1 Inhibitors antagonize the immediate apoptosis triggered by spindle disruption but promote apoptosis following the subsequent rereplication and abnormal mitosis. *Cell Cycle* **2008**, *7*, 1449–1461. [CrossRef]

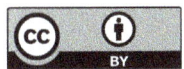

© 2018 by the authors. Licensee MDPI, Basel, Switzerland. This article is an open access article distributed under the terms and conditions of the Creative Commons Attribution (CC BY) license (http://creativecommons.org/licenses/by/4.0/).

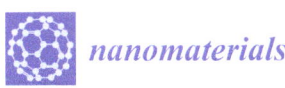

Article

Dose- and Time-Dependent Cytotoxicity of Layered Black Phosphorus in Fibroblastic Cells

Su-Jin Song [1,†], Yong Cheol Shin [2,†], Hyun Uk Lee [3], Bongju Kim [4], Dong-Wook Han [1,*] and Dohyung Lim [5,*]

1. Department of Cogno-Mechatronics Engineering, College of Nanoscience & Nanotechnology, Pusan National University, Busan 46241, Korea; songsj86@gmail.com
2. Research Center for Energy Convergence Technology, Pusan National University, Busan 46241, Korea; choel15@naver.com
3. Advanced Nano-surface Research Group, Korea Basic Science Institute (KBSI), Daejeon 34133, Korea; leeho@kbsi.re.kr
4. Dental Life Science Research Institute, Seoul National University Dental Hospital, Seoul 03080, Korea; bjkim016@gmail.com
5. Department of Mechanical Engineering, Sejong University, Seoul 05006, Korea
* Correspondence: nanohan@pusan.ac.kr (D.-W.H.); dli349@sejong.ac.kr (D.L.); Tel.: +82-51-510-7725 (D.-W.H.); +82-2-3408-3672 (D.L.)
† Those authors contributed equally to this work.

Received: 10 May 2018; Accepted: 4 June 2018; Published: 6 June 2018

Abstract: Black phosphorus (BP) is a monolayer/multilayer two-dimensional (2D) nanomaterial, which has recently emerged as one of the most attractive 2D nanomaterials due to its fascinating physicochemical and optoelectronical properties. Layered BP may have promising applications in biomedical fields, such as drug delivery, photodynamic/photothermal therapy and bioimaging, although its intrinsic toxicity has not been fully elucidated yet. In the present study, the cytotoxicological effects of layered BP on both cell metabolic activity and membrane integrity were investigated. Layered BPs were prepared using a modified ultrasonication-assisted solution method, and their physicochemical properties were characterized. The dose- and time-dependent cytotoxicity of layered BP was assessed against L-929 fibroblasts. Our findings indicate that the cytotoxicity of BPs is proportionally dependent on their concentration and exposure time, which is affected by the oxidative stress-mediated enzyme activity reduction and membrane disruption. On the other hand, layered BPs did not exhibit significant cytotoxicity at concentrations lower than 4 µg/mL. Therefore, it is suggested that layered BPs can be effectively utilized as therapeutic delivery carriers and imaging agents.

Keywords: black phosphorus; 2D nanomaterial; cytotoxicity; biomedical application

1. Introduction

Over the last decade, tremendous research has been conducted to understand and explore the various types of two-dimensional (2D) nanomaterials. This research has found that 2D nanomaterials have a promising potential in a variety of applications, such as optoelectronics, photonics, energy storage and conversion, and biomedicine [1,2]. Among monolayer/multilayer 2D nanomaterials, layered black phosphorus (BP) has recently emerged as an attractive novel one due to its distinct structure, with phosphorenes stacked in several layers via van der Waals forces, and has been acknowledged as one of the most stable allotropes of the phosphorus family [3–8]. Some studies have already shown the potential of BP in biomedical applications, such as drug delivery, photodynamic/photothermal therapy and bioimaging [1,9–13]. However, several controversial results regarding the toxicity of BP have been reported, which means that an in-depth understanding of the cytotoxicity and underlying mechanism of BP is of utmost importance.

A series of studies reported that layered BP has little to no toxic effects, which means that it can be employed as a biomedical material [1,6,13]. It has been found that, while the BPs can induce cell apoptosis and necrosis owing to the transient intracellular reactive oxygen species (ROS)-mediated oxidative stress, the induced oxidative stress can be gradually restored to normal levels with no long-term inflammatory reaction or obvious damage to an in vivo mouse model [14]. Moreover, BP nanosheets can be used as drug delivery vehicles because they have pH- or photo-responsive drug release characteristics as well as a high drug loading efficiency [1,9]. Additionally, BP has been found to possess both outstanding near-infrared photothermal performance and photodynamic activity, which allows it to be utilized for photothermal and photodynamic therapy [9–12,15]. However, although these studies on the biomedical potential of BP could provide valuable guidelines for the essential understanding of the biological effects of BP, the issue of the potential toxicity of BP remains unresolved. In particular, the toxicity of layered BPs is highly varied depending on their concentration, size, shape, surface chemistry, and exposure time, which is similar to the other 2D nanomaterials, such as graphene and its derivatives [14,16,17]. Therefore, prior to the use of layered BP in biomedical applications, it is urgently necessary to investigate its toxicological effects. Hence, in the present study, we assessed the cytotoxicity of layered BP on fibroblastic cells according to its concentration and exposure time, using cytotoxicity assays with different end-points, including the cell metabolic activity, membrane integrity and intracellular ROS production. Our findings revealed that layered BPs showed dose- and time-dependent cytotoxicity, which are caused by oxidative stress-mediated enzyme activity reduction and membrane disruption, but they did not exhibit significant cytotoxicity at a low concentration. These dose- and time-dependent cytotoxicity profiles of layered BPs can be quite informative and useful for their development as biocompatible therapeutic delivery carriers and imaging agents.

2. Materials and Methods

2.1. Preparation and Characterization of Layered BP

Layered BP was prepared by exfoliation of bulk BP crystals using a modified ultrasonication-assisted solution method, as described elsewhere [13]. Fourier transform infrared (FT-IR) spectroscopy was used to characterize the layered BP. The FT-IR spectrum of layered BP was collected using an FT-IR spectroscope (Nicolet Co., Madison, WI, USA) with a resolution of 4.0 cm^{-1} and 16-times scanning in the wavelength range of 750–4000 cm^{-1}. The surface topography of layered BP was analyzed by atomic force microscopy (AFM; NX10, Park Systems Co., Suwon, Korea) in air at room temperature. Imaging was carried out in non-contact mode with a Multi 75 silicon scanning probe at a resonant frequency of ~300 kHz. The average hydrodynamic size of layered BPs was determined using a Zetasizer (Nano ZS, Malvern Instruments, Worcestershire, UK).

2.2. In Vitro Assays for Cytotoxicity Evaluation of Layered BP

L-929 fibroblastic cells were routinely cultured in Dulbecco's modified Eagle's Medium (DMEM, Welgene, Daegu, Korea) supplemented with 10% fetal bovine serum (Welgene) and 1% antibiotic-antimycotic solution (Sigma-Aldrich Co., Saint Louis, MO, USA) at 37 °C in a humidified atmosphere containing 5% CO_2. The cell viability of L-929 cells, treated with layered BP for 24 h, 48 h and 72 h, was assessed by a cell counting kit-8 (CCK-8) assay (Dojindo, Kumamoto, Japan) according to the manufacturer's instructions. Briefly, L-929 fibroblasts were seeded at a density of 1×10^4 cells/mL on a 96-well plate and incubated for 24 h. Subsequently, the cells were treated with various concentrations of layered BP suspended in culture medium (0 to 125 µg/mL) and then incubated with a CCK-8 solution for the last 2 h of the culture period (24 h, 48 h and 72 h) at 37 °C in the dark. The absorbance was measured at 450 nm using an enzyme-linked immunosorbent assay (ELISA) reader (SpectraMax® 340, Molecular Device Co., Sunnyvale, CA, USA). The cell viability was determined to be the percentage ratio of the absorbance values in the cells (incubated with layered BP) to those in untreated control groups (0 µg/mL).

The cell membrane integrity was investigated by monitoring the release of lactate dehydrogenase (LDH) using an LDH assay kit (Takara Bio Inc., Shiga, Japan). After 24 h of incubation with various concentrations of layered BP, the supernatant from each cell culture was transferred to a new 96-well plate. Next, the LDH assay solution was added to each well and then incubated for 30 min at room temperature in the dark. The absorbance was measured at 490 nm using an ELISA reader.

The intracellular ROS production was detected using an ROS assay kit (OxiSelect™; Cell Biolabs, Inc., San Diego, CA, USA). Typically, L-929 cells were plated in a 96-well plate (1×10^4 cells/mL) and incubated for 24 h. The cells were treated with increasing concentrations of layered BP for 24 h. Each cell culture was washed with Dulbecco's phosphate-buffered saline (DPBS, Gibco, Rockville, MD, USA) and then incubated with 2′,7′-dichlorofluororescein diacetate (DCFH-DA), a cell-permeable fluorogenic probe, for 30 min at 37 °C in the dark. The cells were then imaged using an inverted fluorescence microscope (IX81, Olympus, Melville, NY, USA); the fluorescence intensity was determined by a fluorescence plate reader (VICTOR^3 Multilabel Counter, PerkinElmer, Inc., Waltham, MA, USA) with excitation and emission wavelengths of 480 nm and 530 nm, respectively. The fluorescence intensity was expressed as the fold-increase over the values of the untreated control groups.

For morphological observations, the time-lapse images of L-929 cells treated with 10 μg/mL of layered BP were acquired every 1 h for 12 h of incubation. The percentage of live cells was estimated by calculating the ratio of the number of attached cells, defined as cells with a spindle-like morphology (i.e., aspect ratio larger than 1) or specialized subcellular structures, such as lamellipodia, filopodia, stress fibers, and membrane protrusions, to the total number of cells [18–22].

2.3. Statistical Analysis

All variables were tested in three independent cultures for each experiment, which were repeated twice ($n = 6$). All presented data were expressed as average ± standard deviation. Statistical comparisons were carried out by a one-way analysis of variance (SAS Institute Inc., Cary, NC, USA), followed by a Bonferroni test for multiple comparisons. A value of $p < 0.05$ was considered statistically significant.

3. Results and Discussion

3.1. Characteristics of Layered BP

The physicochemical properties of layered BP were characterized by FT-IR spectroscopy and AFM (Figure 1). The FT-IR spectrum of layered BP showed the characteristic peaks of BP crystals (Figure 1a). A noticeable peak was observed near 1000 cm^{-1}, attributed to the stretching vibrations of P–O [23]. The peaks found near 1140 and 1620 cm^{-1} represented the P=O stretching modes of layered BP [23,24]. On the other hand, broad absorption bands were observed, ranging from 2400 cm^{-1} to 3500 cm^{-1}, which could be attributed to the CO_2 stretching and OH stretching vibrations due to exposure of the layered BP to ambient atmosphere. The surface topographic image of layered BP is presented in Figure 1b. Most layered BP were found to have a 2D layer structure, and the average height was about 6.87 ± 0.58 nm (Figure 1b,c). Considering the thickness of the BP monolayer (0.53 nm), the layered BP was composed of several BP monolayers [25]. Moreover, the hydrodynamic size of 2D nanomaterials is of great importance in biomedical applications, because it has a marked effect on the interactions between 2D nanomaterials and cells [17,26–29]. The hydrodynamic size of the BPs used in the present study was found to be 960 ± 303 nm (Figure 1d).

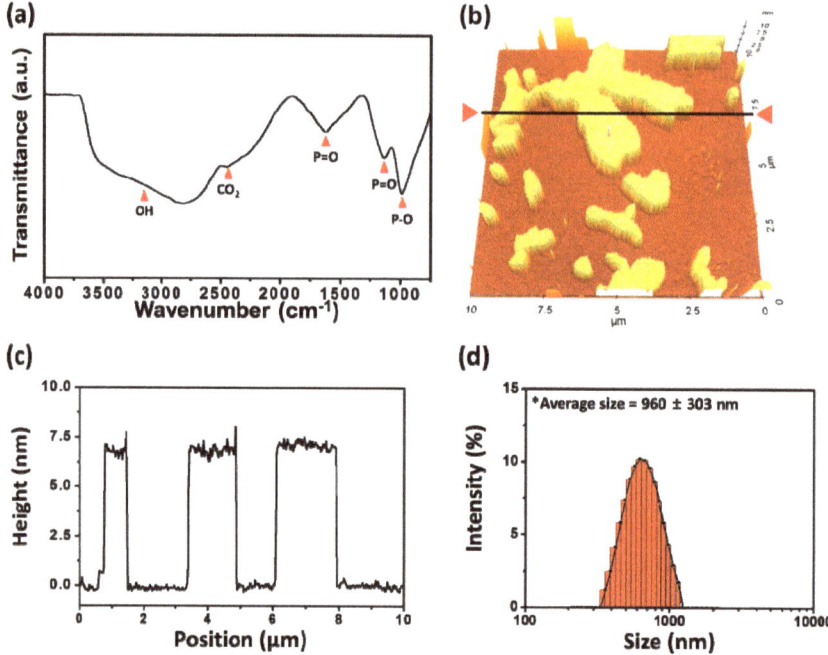

Figure 1. Characterizations of layered BP. (**a**) FT-IR spectrum of layered BP; (**b**) AFM image and (**c**) the height profile of layered BP along the black line marked in (**b**); (**d**) Hydrodynamic size distribution histogram of layered BP.

3.2. Dose-Dependent Cytotoxicity of Layered BP

To investigate the cytotoxic effects of layered BP on L-929 fibroblasts according to its concentration, cells were treated with increasing concentrations of layered BP (0 to 125 µg/mL) for 24 h, and the morphology of the cells was observed (Figure 2a). There were no significant differences in the number and morphology of L-929 fibroblasts at concentrations of up to 4 µg/mL of layered BP. On the other hand, the cells with aggregated BPs exhibited an abnormal morphology and a significant decrease in cell number at concentrations higher than 8 µg/mL, clearly indicating that layered BPs exhibit dose-dependent cytotoxicity. From the CCK-8 assay, based on the cell metabolic activity (Figure 2b), it was found that the cell viability of L-929 fibroblasts decreased as BP concentration increased. At relatively low concentrations (~4 µg/mL), over 82% of fibroblasts were viable, whereas the cell viability of the control at 62 µg/mL decreased to approximately 37%. These findings are inconsistent with previous reports, which found that BP derivatives, including BP nanosheets and nanodots, were nontoxic to several types of cells even when BP concentration was as high as 1000 µg/mL [1,6,9,13]. These conflicting results may be due to size effects. It was demonstrated that layered BPs show a size-dependent cytotoxicity; larger BPs (with lateral size of ~880 nm) were more cytotoxic than smaller ones (with lateral size of ~210 nm) [17]. As shown in Figure 1d, the average lateral size (~960 ± 303 nm) of layered BPs used in this study was relatively larger than that used in other investigations, which can result in greater toxic effects on cells.

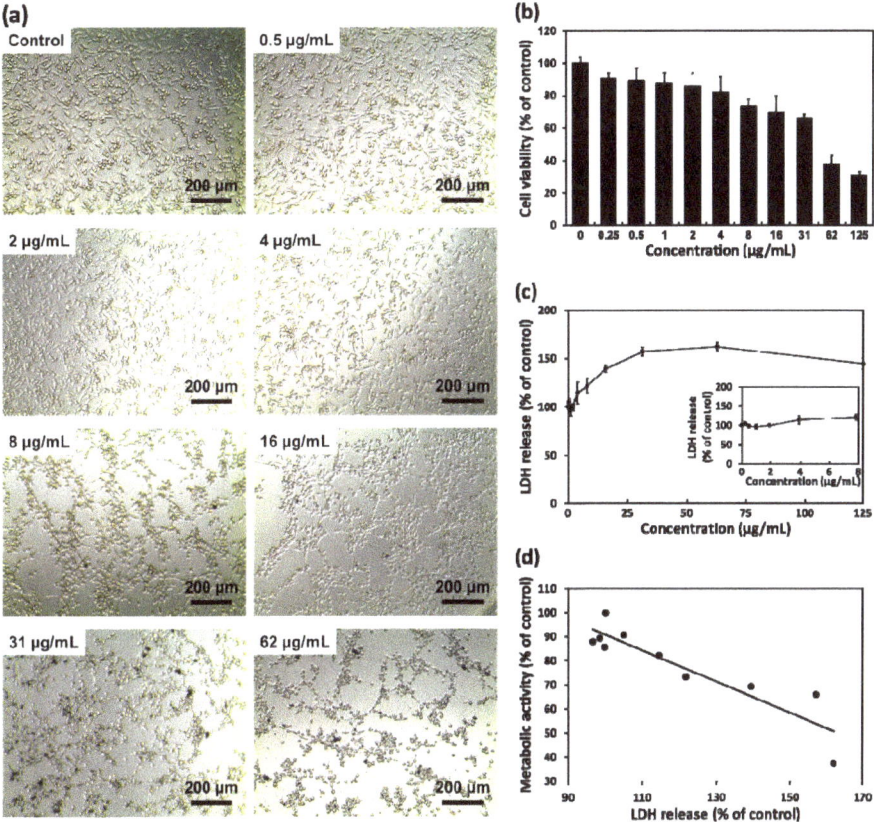

Figure 2. (a) Representative optical microscopy images of L-929 fibroblasts cultured with layered BP (0, 0.5, 2, 4, 8, 16, 31 and 62 μg/mL); (b) Cell viability and (c) LDH release profile of L-929 fibroblasts after 24 h of incubation with various concentrations of layered BP; (d) Correlation coefficient plot between metabolic activity and LDH release for cells cultured with layered BP at concentrations ranging from 0 to 62 μg/mL.

3.3. Membrane Disruption and ROS Production Induced by Layered BP

On the other hand, interesting results were found concerning the cytotoxicity of layered BPs. The cytotoxic effects of layered BPs can be ascribed to membrane disruption [17,30]. Therefore, we investigated the cytotoxicity of layered BPs using LDH assays based on the cell membrane integrity (Figure 2c). The extracellular release of LDH has been extensively used for investigating cell membrane integrity, because LDH, a stable cytoplasmic enzyme, can only be released into extracellular fluids upon plasma membrane disruption [31]. As shown in Figure 2c, a significant LDH release was detected at high concentrations of layered BP ($\geq$16 μg/mL). The LDH release increased to approximately 140% of the control at 16 μg/mL of BP, indicating that high concentrations of layered BPs induced a significant membrane disruption. A slight decrease in LDH release, observed at 125 μg/mL, can be due to the decrease in the total cell number. For CCK-8 and LDH assay results, the calculated value of the corresponding correlation coefficient was -0.91 (Figure 2d), implying that the effects of layered BP on cell metabolic activity and membrane integrity were shown to have a high negative correlation.

At the same time, the dose-dependent cytotoxicity of layered BPs can also be due to oxidative stress. To further investigate the cytotoxicity of layered BPs, the effects of BPs on intracellular ROS generation were evaluated using an ROS-sensitive fluorogenic probe DCFH-DA. The DCFH-DA, a cell-permeable fluorophore, can be readily diffused into cells and subsequently deacetylated by cellular esterases to non-fluorescent DCFH (2′,7′-dichlorodihydrofluorescin). The internalized DCFH is quickly oxidized to highly fluorescent DCF by intracellular ROS. Hence, the intracellular fluorescence of DCF reflects the oxidative stress attributed to the intracellular ROS production. As shown in Figure 3a, the minimal fluorescence was detected at low concentrations of layered BP (≤ 4 µg/mL), while obvious green fluorescence was detected in L-929 cells after incubation with concentrations of layered BP higher than 8 µg/mL. In addition, the fluorescence intensity was significantly ($p < 0.05$) enhanced with increasing concentrations of layered BPs (Figure 3b). It has been documented that the cytotoxicity of BP nanomaterials causes oxidative stress, such as the reduction of enzyme activity, lipid peroxidation and DNA breaks, caused by intracellular ROS production [14]. Thus, even though the size of the layered BP used in the present study was different from that used in previous studies, the cytotoxicity of layered BPs is proportionally dependent on their concentration, which can be attributed to the reduction of metabolic activity owing to oxidative stress. From our in vitro cytotoxicity assay results with different end-points (the cell metabolic activity, membrane integrity and intracellular ROS production), it was revealed that the dose-dependent cytotoxicity of layered BPs was due to both membrane disruption and oxidative stress-mediated metabolic activity reduction.

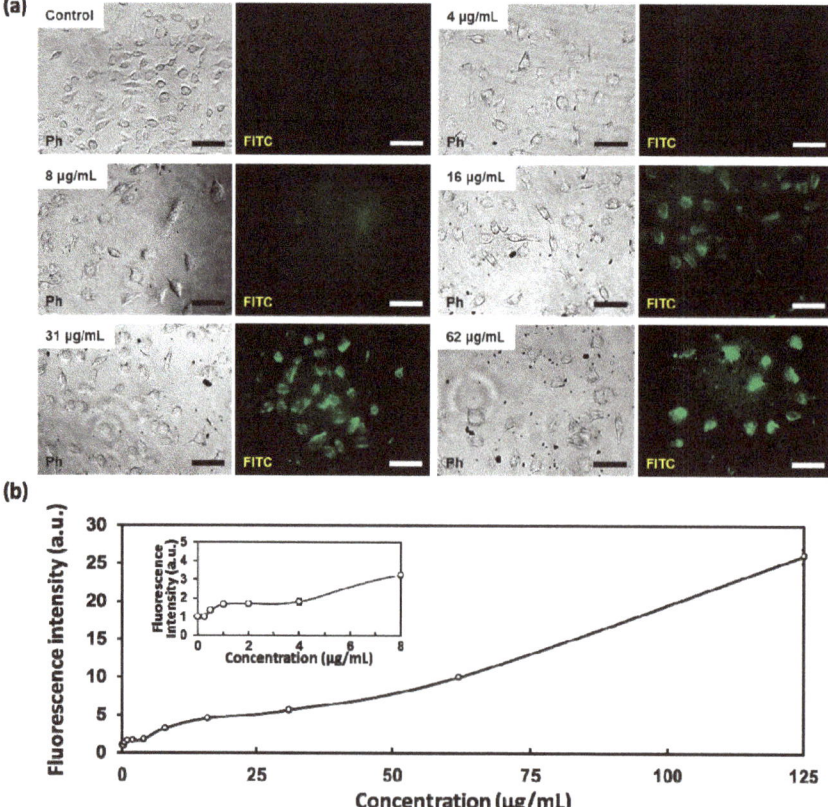

Figure 3. (a) Representative fluorescence microscopy images of oxidized DCF fluorescence in L-929 fibroblasts treated with various concentrations of layered BP (0, 4, 8, 16, 31 and 62 µg/mL) for 24 h; and (b) quantification of oxidized DCF fluorescence intensity. The scale bars are 100 µm.

3.4. Time-Dependent Cytotoxicity of Layered BP

To further evaluate the toxic effects of layered BPs on cells, we observed the morphological changes of L-929 fibroblasts and estimated the number of live cells. The time-lapse images of cells, treated with 10 µg/mL of layered BP for an initial 12 h at an interval of 1 h, are shown in Figure 4a. The number of live cells was estimated by quantifying the ratio of the number of attached cells to the total number of cells (Figure 4b). Because adherent cells, including fibroblastic cells, have to be attached to appropriate substrates in order to survive, the cells, which did not show typical fibroblastic morphology, were considered to be dead [18–22]. It was observed that the number of cells with apoptotic morphology (marked in red) increased throughout incubation with layered BPs for the initial 12 h (Figure 4a). In particular, the live cells decreased significantly ($p < 0.05$) after 6 h of incubation with layered BPs (Figure 4b). The morphological changes were clearly observed by comparing optical microscopy images, taken every hour for 12 h (Figure 4c). These results implied that the cytotoxicity of layered BPs is also dependent on their exposure time.

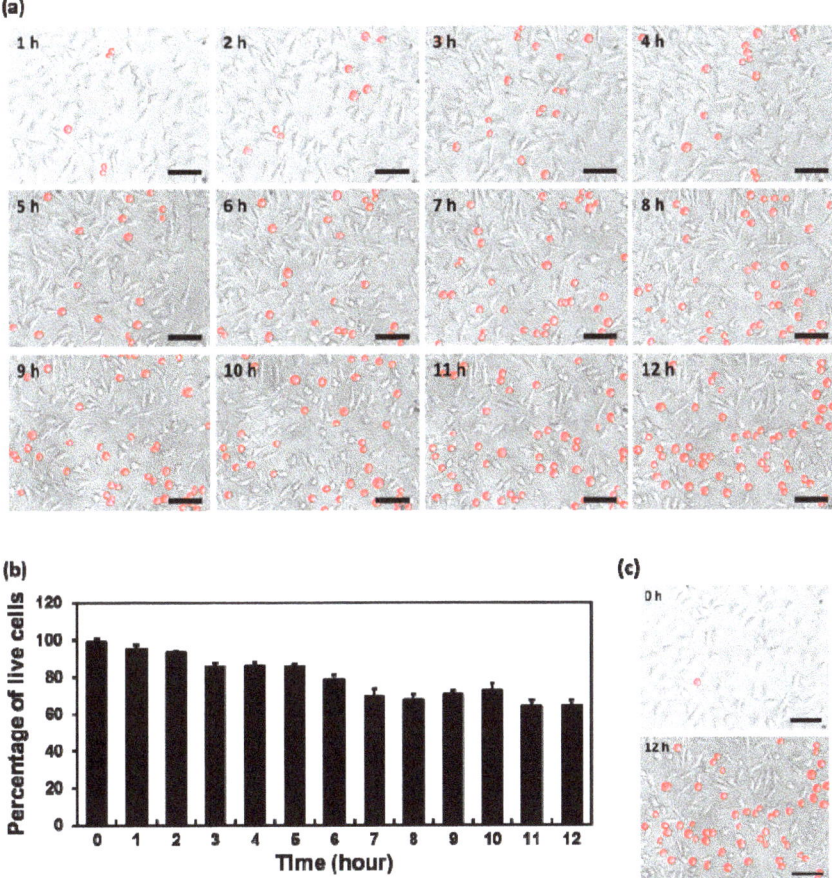

Figure 4. (a) Time-lapse images of L-929 cells treated with 10 µg/mL of layered BP for an initial 12 h at an interval of 1 h; (b) Quantification of the percentage of live cells for 12 h; (c) Optical microscopy images of L-929 fibroblasts treated with 10 µg/mL of layered BP for 0 and 12 h. The scale bars are 100 µm.

The cell viability of L-929 fibroblasts, incubated with layered BP for 48 and 72 h, was evaluated to further examine the time-dependent cytotoxicity of layered BP, as shown in Figure 5a,b, respectively. The cytotoxic effects of layered BPs after 48 and 72 h are also dose-dependent, which is similar to the results after 24 h. Additionally, the cell viability after 48 and 72 h decreased more than it did after 24 h, as the incubation time with layered BPs had increased, and the decrease in cell viability after 72 h was more significant than after 48 h. At a concentration of 16 µg/mL, the cell viability after 48 and 72 h decreased to approximately 60% and 45% of the control, respectively. These results indicated that the cytotoxic effects of layered BPs were also dependent on exposure time. Consequently, it was revealed that the layered BP exhibited dose- and time-dependent cytotoxicity, as a result of membrane disruption and oxidative stress-mediated metabolic activity reduction caused by the accumulation of intracellular ROS as well as the interactions between layered BPs and cells. However, it is worth noting that the layered BPs were not significantly cytotoxic at concentrations lower than 4 µg/mL, suggesting that layered BPs in the range of only a few µg/mL can be effectively used in biomedical applications, such as therapeutic delivery carriers and imaging agents. Furthermore, to improve biocompatibility and biological activity, BPs can be conjugated or modified with various functional compounds, such as biocompatible polymers, nanoparticles and drugs [1,10,12,15]. It has been revealed that the encapsulation of BPs with poly(lactic-co-glycolic acid), a biodegradable polymer, allows not only the enhancement of biocompatibility, but also the degradation of nontoxic phosphate and phosphonate [12]. These results indicated that, although the cytotoxicity of BPs is closely dependent on their concentration and exposure time, the BPs with the desirable modification can be compatibly employed in biomedical applications, even at concentrations higher than 8 µg/mL. In summary, it is suggested that BP has a promising potential as a biomedical material.

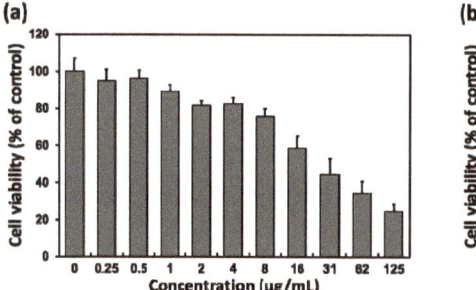
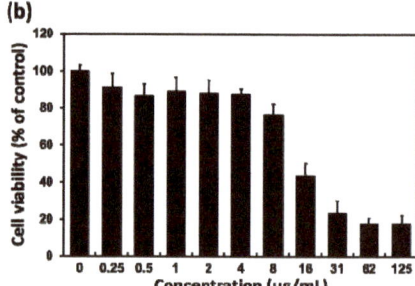

Figure 5. Cell viability profiles of L-929 fibroblasts after (**a**) 48 and (**b**) 72 h of incubation with various concentrations of layered BP.

4. Conclusions

This study aimed to investigate the dose- and time-dependent cytotoxicity of layered BPs against L-929 fibroblasts. It was revealed that the cytotoxicity of layered BPs was proportionally dependent on their concentration and exposure time. These cytotoxic effects of layered BPs are found to be due to both oxidative stress-mediated enzyme activity reduction and membrane disruption. On the other hand, the cytotoxicity of layered BPs is not significant at concentrations lower than 4 µg/mL. Taken together, this work suggests that layered BPs can be effectively used in biomedical applications, such as therapeutic delivery carriers and imaging agents, although further comprehensive studies are undoubtedly necessary to fundamentally explore and understand the more detailed mechanisms behind the toxic effects of BPs.

Author Contributions: S.-J.S. and Y.C.S. designed the experiments, performed the in vitro assays and drafted the manuscript. H.U.L. carried out the preparation and characterization of layered BPs. B.K. performed the statistical analysis and helped to interpret the data. D.-W.H. and D.L. conceived of the study, participated in its design and coordination, and helped to draft the manuscript. All authors read and approved the final manuscript.

Funding: This work was supported by a 2-year research grant from Pusan National University.

Conflicts of Interest: The authors declare no conflict of interest.

References

1. Tao, W.; Zhu, X.; Yu, X.; Zeng, X.; Xiao, Q.; Zhang, X.; Ji, X.; Wang, X.; Shi, J.; Zhang, H. Black phosphorus nanosheets as a robust delivery platform for cancer theranostics. *Adv. Mater.* **2017**, *29*, 1603276. [CrossRef] [PubMed]
2. Shin, Y.C.; Song, S.-J.; Hong, S.W.; Jeong, S.J.; Chrzanowski, W.; Lee, J.-C.; Han, D.-W. Multifaceted biomedical applications of functional graphene nanomaterials to coated substrates, patterned arrays and hybrid scaffolds. *Nanomaterials* **2017**, *7*, 369. [CrossRef] [PubMed]
3. Chen, Y.; Ren, R.; Pu, H.; Chang, J.; Mao, S.; Chen, J. Field-effect transistor biosensors with two-dimensional black phosphorus nanosheets. *Biosens. Bioelectron.* **2017**, *89*, 505–510. [CrossRef] [PubMed]
4. Li, C.; Xie, Z.; Chen, Z.; Cheng, N.; Wang, J.; Zhu, G. Tunable bandgap and optical properties of black phosphorene nanotubes. *Materials* **2018**, *11*, 304. [CrossRef] [PubMed]
5. Xia, F.; Wang, H.; Jia, Y. Rediscovering black phosphorus as an anisotropic layered material for optoelectronics and electronics. *Nat. Commun.* **2014**, *5*, 4458. [CrossRef] [PubMed]
6. Engel, M.; Steiner, M.; Avouris, P. Black phosphorus photodetector for multispectral, high-resolution imaging. *Nano Lett.* **2014**, *14*, 6414–6417. [CrossRef] [PubMed]
7. Lee, T.H.; Kim, S.Y.; Jang, H.W. Black phosphorus: Critical review and potential for water splitting photocatalyst. *Nanomaterials* **2016**, *6*, 194. [CrossRef] [PubMed]
8. Jiang, X.-F.; Zeng, Z.; Li, S.; Guo, Z.; Zhang, H.; Huang, F.; Xu, Q.-H. Tunable broadband nonlinear optical properties of black phosphorus quantum dots for femtosecond laser pulses. *Materials* **2017**, *10*, 210. [CrossRef] [PubMed]
9. Chen, W.; Ouyang, J.; Liu, H.; Chen, M.; Zeng, K.; Sheng, J.; Liu, Z.; Han, Y.; Wang, L.; Li, J. Black phosphorus nanosheet-based drug delivery system for synergistic photodynamic/photothermal/chemotherapy of cancer. *Adv. Mater.* **2017**, *29*, 1603864. [CrossRef] [PubMed]
10. Sun, Z.; Xie, H.; Tang, S.; Yu, X.F.; Guo, Z.; Shao, J.; Zhang, H.; Huang, H.; Wang, H.; Chu, P.K. Ultrasmall black phosphorus quantum dots: Synthesis and use as photothermal agents. *Angew. Chem.* **2015**, *127*, 11688–11692. [CrossRef]
11. Wang, H.; Yang, X.; Shao, W.; Chen, S.; Xie, J.; Zhang, X.; Wang, J.; Xie, Y. Ultrathin black phosphorus nanosheets for efficient singlet oxygen generation. *J. Am. Chem. Soc.* **2015**, *137*, 11376–11382. [CrossRef] [PubMed]
12. Shao, J.; Xie, H.; Huang, H.; Li, Z.; Sun, Z.; Xu, Y.; Xiao, Q.; Yu, X.-F.; Zhao, Y.; Zhang, H. Biodegradable black phosphorus-based nanospheres for in vivo photothermal cancer therapy. *Nat. Commun.* **2016**, *7*, 12967. [CrossRef] [PubMed]
13. Lee, H.U.; Park, S.Y.; Lee, S.C.; Choi, S.; Seo, S.; Kim, H.; Won, J.; Choi, K.; Kang, K.S.; Park, H.G. Black phosphorus (BP) nanodots for potential biomedical applications. *Small* **2016**, *12*, 214–219. [CrossRef] [PubMed]
14. Mu, X.; Wang, J.-Y.; Bai, X.; Xu, F.; Liu, H.; Yang, J.; Jing, Y.; Liu, L.; Xue, X.; Dai, H. Black phosphorus quantum dot induced oxidative stress and toxicity in living cells and mice. *ACS Appl. Mater. Interfaces* **2017**, *9*, 20399–20409. [CrossRef] [PubMed]
15. Lv, R.; Yang, D.; Yang, P.; Xu, J.; He, F.; Gai, S.; Li, C.; Dai, Y.; Yang, G.; Lin, J. Integration of upconversion nanoparticles and ultrathin black phosphorus for efficient photodynamic theranostics under 808 nm near-infrared light irradiation. *Chem. Mater.* **2016**, *28*, 4724–4734. [CrossRef]
16. Latiff, N.M.; Teo, W.Z.; Sofer, Z.; Fisher, A.C.; Pumera, M. The cytotoxicity of layered black phosphorus. *Chem. Eur. J.* **2015**, *21*, 13991–13995. [CrossRef] [PubMed]
17. Zhang, X.; Zhang, Z.; Zhang, S.; Li, D.; Ma, W.; Ma, C.; Wu, F.; Zhao, Q.; Yan, Q.; Xing, B. Size effect on the cytotoxicity of layered black phosphorus and underlying mechanisms. *Small* **2017**, *13*, 1701210. [CrossRef] [PubMed]

18. Kimmel, K.A.; Carey, T.E. Altered expression in squamous carcinoma cells of an orientation restricted epithelial antigen detected by monoclonal antibody A9. *Cancer Res.* **1986**, *46*, 3614–3623. [PubMed]
19. Giancotti, F.G.; Ruoslahti, E. Integrin signaling. *Science* **1999**, *285*, 1028–1033. [CrossRef] [PubMed]
20. Tseng, Y.; Kole, T.P.; Lee, S.-H.J.; Wirtz, D. Local dynamics and viscoelastic properties of cell biological systems. *Curr. Opin. Colloid Interface Sci.* **2002**, *7*, 210–217. [CrossRef]
21. Hood, J.D.; Cheresh, D.A. Role of integrins in cell invasion and migration. *Nat. Rev. Cancer* **2002**, *2*, 91–100. [CrossRef] [PubMed]
22. Jin, H.; Pi, J.; Huang, X.; Huang, F.; Shao, W.; Li, S.; Chen, Y.; Cai, J. BMP2 promotes migration and invasion of breast cancer cells via cytoskeletal reorganization and adhesion decrease: An AFM investigation. *Appl. Microbiol. Biotechnol.* **2012**, *93*, 1715–1723. [CrossRef] [PubMed]
23. Sun, C.; Wen, L.; Zeng, J.; Wang, Y.; Sun, Q.; Deng, L.; Zhao, C.; Li, Z. One-pot solventless preparation of PEGylated black phosphorus nanoparticles for photoacoustic imaging and photothermal therapy of cancer. *Biomaterials* **2016**, *91*, 81–89. [CrossRef] [PubMed]
24. Ge, S.; Zhang, L.; Wang, P.; Fang, Y. Intense, stable and excitation wavelength-independent photoluminescence emission in the blue-violet region from phosphorene quantum dots. *Sci. Rep.* **2016**, *6*, 27307. [CrossRef] [PubMed]
25. Wang, X.; Jones, A.M.; Seyler, K.L.; Tran, V.; Jia, Y.; Zhao, H.; Wang, H.; Yang, L.; Xu, X.; Xia, F. Highly anisotropic and robust excitons in monolayer black phosphorus. *Nat. Nanotechnol.* **2015**, *10*, 517–521. [CrossRef] [PubMed]
26. Mahmoudi, M.; Simchi, A.; Milani, A.S.; Stroeve, P. Cell toxicity of superparamagnetic iron oxide nanoparticles. *J. Colloid Interface Sci.* **2009**, *336*, 510–518. [CrossRef] [PubMed]
27. Chang, Y.; Yang, S.-T.; Liu, J.-H.; Dong, E.; Wang, Y.; Cao, A.; Liu, Y.; Wang, H. In vitro toxicity evaluation of graphene oxide on A549 cells. *Toxicol. Lett.* **2011**, *200*, 201–210. [CrossRef] [PubMed]
28. Akhavan, O.; Ghaderi, E.; Akhavan, A. Size-dependent genotoxicity of graphene nanoplatelets in human stem cells. *Biomaterials* **2012**, *33*, 8017–8025. [CrossRef] [PubMed]
29. Ma, J.; Liu, R.; Wang, X.; Liu, Q.; Chen, Y.; Valle, R.P.; Zuo, Y.Y.; Xia, T.; Liu, S. Crucial role of lateral size for graphene oxide in activating macrophages and stimulating pro-inflammatory responses in cells and animals. *ACS Nano* **2015**, *9*, 10498–10515. [CrossRef] [PubMed]
30. Hu, W.; Peng, C.; Lv, M.; Li, X.; Zhang, Y.; Chen, N.; Fan, C.; Huang, Q. Protein corona-mediated mitigation of cytotoxicity of graphene oxide. *ACS Nano* **2011**, *5*, 3693–3700. [CrossRef] [PubMed]
31. Schneider, Y.; Chabert, P.; Stutzmann, J.; Coelho, D.; Fougerousse, A.; Gossé, F.; Launay, J.F.; Brouillard, R.; Raul, F. Resveratrol analog (Z)-3,5,4'-trimethoxystilbene is a potent anti-mitotic drug inhibiting tubulin polymerization. *Int. J. Cancer* **2003**, *107*, 189–196. [CrossRef] [PubMed]

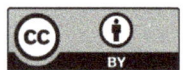

© 2018 by the authors. Licensee MDPI, Basel, Switzerland. This article is an open access article distributed under the terms and conditions of the Creative Commons Attribution (CC BY) license (http://creativecommons.org/licenses/by/4.0/).

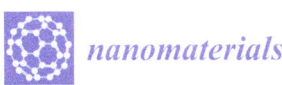

Review

ZnO Nanostructures and Electrospun ZnO–Polymeric Hybrid Nanomaterials in Biomedical, Health, and Sustainability Applications

Eloisa Ferrone [1], Rodolfo Araneo [1,*], Andrea Notargiacomo [2], Marialilia Pea [2] and Antonio Rinaldi [3,*]

1. Department of Electrical Engineering, University of Rome Sapienza, 00184 Rome, Italy; eloisa.ferrone@gmail.com
2. Institute for Photonics and Nanotechnologies–CNR, 00156 Rome, Italy; andrea.notargiacomo@ifn.cnr.it (A.N.); marialilia.pea@ifn.cnr.it (M.P.)
3. Sustainability Department, ENEA, C.R. Casaccia, Santa Maria di Galeria, Rome 00123, Italy
* Correspondence: rodolfo.araneo@uniroma1.it (R.A.); antonio.rinaldi@enea.it (A.R.)

Received: 10 September 2019; Accepted: 3 October 2019; Published: 12 October 2019

Abstract: ZnO-based nanomaterials are a subject of increasing interest within current research, because of their multifunctional properties, such as piezoelectricity, semi-conductivity, ultraviolet absorption, optical transparency, and photoluminescence, as well as their low toxicity, biodegradability, low cost, and versatility in achieving diverse shapes. Among the numerous fields of application, the use of nanostructured ZnO is increasingly widespread also in the biomedical and healthcare sectors, thanks to its antiseptic and antibacterial properties, role as a promoter in tissue regeneration, selectivity for specific cell lines, and drug delivery function, as well as its electrochemical and optical properties, which make it a good candidate for biomedical applications. Because of its growing use, understanding the toxicity of ZnO nanomaterials and their interaction with biological systems is crucial for manufacturing relevant engineering materials. In the last few years, ZnO nanostructures were also used to functionalize polymer matrices to produce hybrid composite materials with new properties. Among the numerous manufacturing methods, electrospinning is becoming a mainstream technique for the production of scaffolds and mats made of polymeric and metal-oxide nanofibers. In this review, we focus on toxicological aspects and recent developments in the use of ZnO-based nanomaterials for biomedical, healthcare, and sustainability applications, either alone or loaded inside polymeric matrices to make electrospun composite nanomaterials. Bibliographic data were compared and analyzed with the aim of giving homogeneity to the results and highlighting reference trends useful for obtaining a fresh perspective about the toxicity of ZnO nanostructures and their underlying mechanisms for the materials and engineering community.

Keywords: ZnO nanostructures; toxicity; biocompatibility; physicochemical properties; cells viability assays; in vivo experiments

---

1. Introduction

In recent decades, zinc oxide (ZnO) became an extremely popular in material science because of its multifunctional properties, low cost, and great versatility of use in various research areas and applications. The scientific interest was accompanied by a considerable growth of the ZnO market in industry, in sectors such as rubber, ceramic materials [1,2], paints [3,4], food packaging [5], cosmetics, and pharmaceutical products [6,7], as well as being highly used for electronic devices [8]. In addition, ZnO is recognized as a bio-safe material, and its use in cosmetic products is approved by the Food and Drug Administration (FDA), which is certainly a driving force in ZnO market growth. ZnO becomes all the more interesting in nanostructured form (i.e., shapes with at least one characteristic dimension less than 100 nm), enabling the realization of novel nanomaterials and nanodevices with special chemical–physical properties [9]. Moreover, it has the great advantage of easy synthesis with various techniques to achieve a vast group of nanostructures (NStr) including nanoparticles (NPs), nanowires (NWs), nanofibers (NFs), nanoflowers (NFls), nanorods (NRs), nanosheets (NSs), nanotubes (NTs), nanoribbons (NRBs), and tetrapods (TPs) [10–14], which suit best different given applications. The main application areas of nanostructured ZnO, summarized in Figure 1, range from electronics (with particular reference to flexible applications) to renewable energy and batteries, building materials, catalysts, and, not least, sustainability and biomedical applications. In fact, the use of nanostructured ZnO is highly increasing in the biomedical and healthcare sectors, allowing for diverse applications including antibacterial materials [15], tissue-engineering scaffolds [16], wound healing [17], drug delivery [18], molecular biosensors [19], and fluorescence imaging [20].

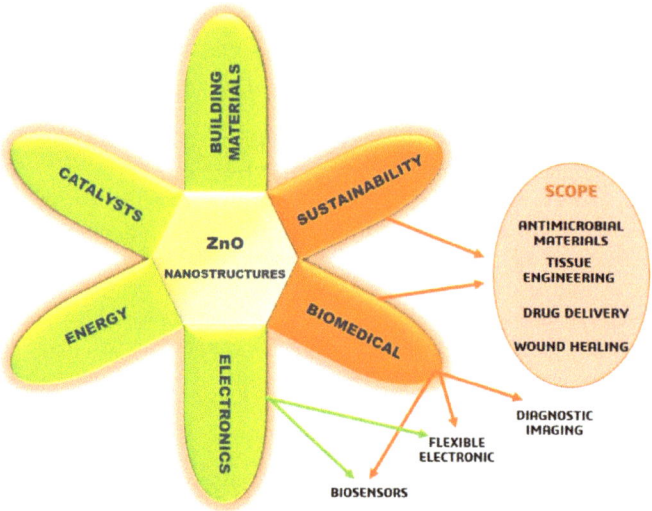

Figure 1. Applications of ZnO nanostructures, focusing on biomedical health and sustainability.

Since ZnO nanostructures are biologically very active because they can produce reactive oxygen species (ROS) and release Zn^{2+} ions [21], the development of new ZnO-based nanomaterials is indeed always accompanied by toxicological studies to test their biocompatibility. While still an open subject of research, numerous studies showed that the use of small amounts of ZnO NStr promotes cell growth, proliferation, and differentiation, as well as tissue regeneration, boosting angiogenesis and osteointegration processes, further supported by ZnO antibacterial and antifungal properties [22–24]. Moreover, ZnO NStr also present selectivity with respect to particular cell lines, which makes them potential candidates for killing cancer cells [25]. In addition to toxicological issues, the relationship between ZnO-based systems (materials and nanocomposites) and biological microenvironments is also particularly relevant for diverse target applications, as summarized in Figure 2, such that much effort is required at the materials design and manufacturing stage to ensure safe and effective application.

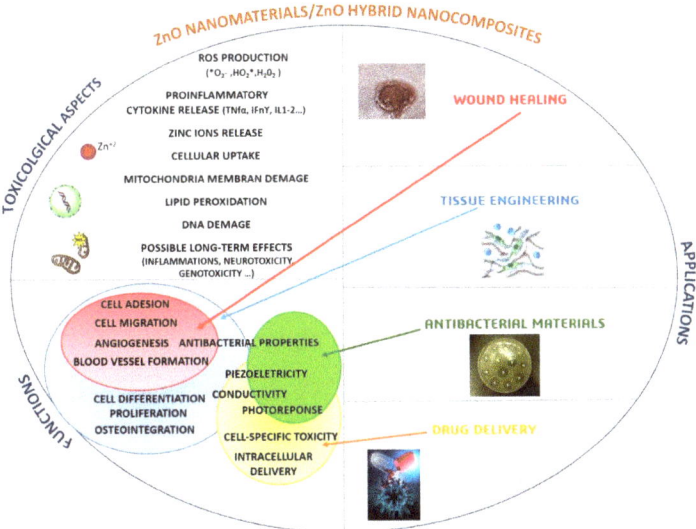

Figure 2. Toxicological aspects, functions, and scope of applications of ZnO-based nanomaterials and ZnO hybrid nanocomposites.

Within the manufacturing processes of novel biomaterials based on ZnO NStr, numerous methodologies use polymer matrices filled with metal oxides, to create high-performance hybrid composite materials [26,27]. Electrospinning is perhaps the most versatile and promising of these techniques, with low cost, ease of processing, and high scalability, which allows achieving two- and three-dimensional (2D and 3D) scaffolds of micro- and nanofibers [28]. This method makes it possible to produce large-scale continuous nanofibers which can be suitably set by acting on the process parameters [29]. The electrospinning technique allows the production of materials with controlled porosity and a large surface-to-volume ratio, which form an interconnected network suitable for biological applications, thanks to their morphological and mechanical properties [30]. The ZnO NStr can be used as fillers inside the electrospun polymer matrix or can be synthesized by post-processing polymer fibers, using hydrothermal processes or other techniques [31,32]. Finally, it is also possible to fabricate ZnO fibers by calcining the material after electrospinning process [33]. Biological processes are strongly influenced by material parameters such as fiber diameter, degree of porosity, shape and interconnection of pores, topography of the surfaces, homogeneity of dispersion of filling elements, and their concentration [34]. All these aspects can be appropriately set and monitored by acting on the electrospinning process parameters [35]. By combining the properties of the nanostructured ZnO with the ease of fabrication of the electrospinning technique, it is possible to develop innovative high-performance materials for many applications [36–38].

While many recent results about ZnO nanostructures and ZnO–polymeric nanocomposites manufactured by electrospinning exist for biomedical, health, and sustainability applications, the literature appears fragmented, and there is a need to critically investigate data trends and possible contradictions in the experimental data to boost further development in materials design and engineering.

In this review, we focus on the use of nanostructured ZnO, both alone and within hybrid composite polymeric materials produced by electrospinning, for biomedical and sustainability applications. In Sections 2 and 3, we reconsider the results of recent studies (in vitro and in vivo) on ZnO-based nanostructures with the aim of pointing out the underlying toxicity mechanisms, a preliminary aspect of fundamental importance for any safe deployment in engineering applications for life and environment. In Section 4, we report the synthesis approaches used for obtaining biosafe ZnO nanostructures for biomedical applications. Section 5 puts a spotlight on the influence of the chemical and physical properties of the ZnO nanostructures. Finally, in Section 6, we focus on ZnO–polymeric hybrid electrospun nanomaterials. Noteworthy, the effects of process parameters in electrospinning, such as different solvents, flow rates, needle-collector distance, etc., on fiber morphology and, to a certain extent, on biological performance are not in the scope of this review.

2. Toxicity Studies on ZnO Nanostructures In Vitro

In this section, we report the main toxicity issues raised in the literature about ZnO nanostructures, as preliminary content for the subsequent survey of results and discussion later in this paper. We split the review and discussion into two subsections according to the presence of a large amount of data present on ZnO NPs which are considered first, before moving to other kinds of ZnO NStr.

2.1. ZnO Nanoparticles

The widespread use of ZnO NPs in many sectors was already highlighted; however, there are still open issues about their interaction mechanisms with biological systems, making this aspect still the object of study and research [39]. Hanley et al. [40] showed that ZnO nanoparticles induce a different cytotoxic response in primary human immune peripheral blood mononuclear cells (PBMC). In particular they found that lymphocytes are the most resistant cells, while monocytes are the most sensitive. All lymphocyte populations (cluster of differentiation 3-positive T cells (T-CD3), T-CD4, B) have a similar half maximal inhibitory concentration value (IC_{50}; the concentration of drug/substance that is require for 50% inhibition in vitro) to all nanoparticle concentrations, while natural killer cells (NK) are more sensitive and show significant statistical differences at concentrations ranging from 1 to 5 mM; monocytes were even more sensitive with a mortality rate above 50% even at the lowest concentrations. It is important, in this regard, to consider the influence of physiological factors such as the electrostatic interaction between cell and nanoparticle, as well as intrinsic differences in the endocytosis/phagocytosis process. Other differences were found between native lymphocytes and memory lymphocytes, which could be linked to the fact that this second type of cells requires a lower level of activation of the threshold signal for proliferation, partly due to changes in the calcium level at the intracellular level. They also investigated the relationship between nanoparticle size and ROS production. What emerged is that cytotoxicity is inversely proportional to the size, with nanoparticles of 4 nm presenting the highest concentration of ROS value. Finally, they focused on the mechanisms of induction of immunoregulatory cytokines, a relevant factor to be considered for the potential use of ZnO NPs in biomedical applications. Their results showed that the induction of interferon gamma (IFN-γ), tumor necrosis factor alpha (TFN-α), and interleukin 12 (IL-12) is concentration-dependent, which is consistent with the production of oxidative stress and inflammation. This aspect indicates that the administration of ZnO NPs can elevate the production of important cytokines to stimulate a local response for an effective anti-tumor action. However, the potential damage from prolonged exposure to these cytokines should not be ignored and, hence, it is fundamental to control parameters such as size, concentration, and biodistribution of nanoparticles for their use in biomedical applications.

In other studies, Hanley and co-workers [41] showed that ZnO NPs induce cell-specific and proliferation-dependent toxicity, observing that rapidly dividing cells are more susceptible to ZnO toxicity with respect to quiescent ones. They highlighted the effects on tumor Jurkat cells and normal primary T-cells belonging to the same cell lineage and showed the differences between activated and resting T lymphocytes. The results showed that cancerous lymphocytes are about 25 to 35 times more susceptible to ZnO NPs than their normal counterparts. For this reason, the NPs can be designed to bind with antibodies, peptides, or small protein molecules associated with tumors, or they can be used for drug delivery. Moreover, the possibility of selectively eliminating activated T cells can be used for the treatment of autoimmune diseases such as multiple sclerosis and psoriasis, in which self-reactive T cells are one of the main groups underlying pathogenic processes. The inactivated state of these cells is verified by the lack of cluster of differentiation 40 L (CD40 L), a marker for T-cell activation.

Finally, ROS production from PBMCs exposed to different concentrations of ZnO NPs and at different exposure times was investigated. Among these, monocyte cells ranked higher in the production of ROS. To evaluate the link between cell mortality and ROS production, T cells were pre-treated with N-acetylcysteine (NAC), a known ROS quencher. What emerged was that the use of NAC contributes significantly to preventing toxicity from ZnO NPs, indicating that the generation of ROS plays an important role in the toxicity induced by nanoparticles.

In the study by Heng et al. [42], the effects of spherical and sheet-like ZnO NPs on RAW-264.7 murine macrophages, BEAS-2B human bronchial epithelial cells, and mouse dendritic primitive cells (DC) were compared. Their choice to use human bronchial epithelial cells stemmed from the fact that the respiratory apparatus is often the first to come into contact with the polluted environment. Macrophages, on the other hand, are important components of the immune system, and it is, therefore, appropriate to study their interaction with the nanoparticles. Exposure of DC cells to ZnO NPs upregulates the expression of cluster of differentiation 80 (CD80) and cluster of differentiation 86 (CD86), known markers of DC activation and maturation, and stimulates the release of proinflammatory cytokines interleukin 6 (IL-6) and TNF-α, an aspect that emphasizes the potential role of ZnO NPs in inducing inflammation. For the experiments, spherical NPs and sheet-like NPs, with an average size of 20×20 nm and 325×15 nm, respectively, and concentration ranging from 1 to 30 µg/mL, were used. The results indicated a strongly dose-dependent behavior. The RAW-264.7 cell line appeared statistically more sensitive to spheriform particles than the BEAS-2B line, especially at high concentrations. This increased sensitivity may indicate that the cytotoxicity mechanism of ZnO NPs may involve the process of phagocytosis, or a second explanation could be that the ZnO NPs bind particular receptors of RAW-264.7 and activate apoptotic pathways. The differences in the cytotoxicity of the two forms could instead be due to differences in the dissolution rate. In any case, both forms stimulate the production of TNF-α with levels up to 200 times higher than the control, even at low concentrations (0.3 µg/mL). Finally, the associations of the ZnO NPs with both cell lines were evaluated, and the greater association occurred with the spherical nanoparticles, probably due to their smaller size. Moreover, the association was maximum after 4 h and then decreased. One root cause could be the process of exocytosis of the NPs after they are absorbed and accumulated inside the cells. The increased association of spherical NPs could make them more suitable for anti-tumor and drug delivery applications.

The same research group studied the cytotoxicity of ZnO NPs in BEAS-2B cells, highlighting the influence of oxidative stress in aggravating cytotoxic effects [43]. In that study, the cells were pre-exposed to 5 and 10 µM H_2O_2 for 45 min and subsequently exposed to variable concentrations of ZnO NPs with a size of about 10 nm. The results demonstrated an increase in cytotoxicity for cells pre-exposed to H_2O_2 with significant differences between those exposed to concentrations of 5 µM and those at 10 µM. The vitality test was not performed immediately, but 24 h later, as the activation of apoptotic pathways took some time to occur. It is to be noted that the cells exposed only to ZnO NPs had values of viability above 99% up to 10 µg/mL NP concentration, which then collapsed rapidly once exceeding this value. These data suggest the existence of a threshold value for the concentration of nanoparticles that does not compromise cell viability, a value that, however, decreases significantly in the presence of oxidative stress.

Wang et al. [44] studied the effects of toxicity and related action mechanisms on RAW 264.7 macrophage cells, in terms of cell viability, MTT (3-(4,5-dimethylthiazol-2-yl)-2,5-diphenyltetrazolium bromide) tetrazolium reduction assay, a colorimetric assay for assessing cell metabolic activity, mitochondrial membrane potential (MMP), total and released lactate dehydrogenase activity (LDH), intracellular ROS level, and Zn^{2+} ion concentration. The ZnO NPs were characterized in terms of morphology, size, surface charge, and solubility. The NPs had a polyhedral shape with an average diameter of about 37 nm. The average size in water was about 229 nm, according to the dynamic light scattering (DLS) measures, and, in some cases, there were aggregation phenomena due to a lack of surface protection. On the surface, they had a slight negative charge of −16 mV. In Dulbecco's modified Eagle medium (DMEM), the dimensions increased significantly (about 1080 nm) due to the presence of salts that shielded the charge repulsion, allowing greater aggregation. Finally, in DMEM supplemented with 10% fetal bovine serum (FBS), there was a reduction in size (800 nm) due to the absorption of serum proteins, allowing a greater stabilization of the particles, in addition to a zeta potential increase to about −9 mV. Solubility studies at different pH values were performed to analyze the release of Zn^{2+} ions. What was found is that the release of ions in an acidic cell culture medium, namely, a phosphate-buffered saline (PBS) with 10% FBS (pH 5.5) that can be considered a lysosomal-mimicking medium, was of an order of magnitude greater than the value achieved in a culture medium at pH 7.2 (DMEM with 10% FBS). This result, in the authors' opinion, is deemed reasonable because the acidic environment reached in these organelles releases H^+ ions, which react easily with the ZnO to form Zn^{2+} and H_2O. Cell viability studies showed time- and dose-dependent cytotoxicity, with decreasing viability as the NP concentration and incubation time increased. The study was performed for concentrations of ZnO NPs ranging from 25 to 200 µg/mL and incubation times of 4, 12, 24, and 48 h. The LDH activity was also measured. Those results were consistent with the MTT test, with LDH release increasing as incubation time increased, suggesting that cell membrane rupture is among the major causes of cytotoxicity. The MMP test was performed as an indicator of mitochondrial activity. MMP values of cells incubated with ZnO NPs decreased with incubation time, but at a faster rate than LDH values, which indicates that mitochondrial function is more compromised than cellular integrity. Finally, the concentration levels of intracellular Zn^{2+} and ROS were measured. There is still reason for uncertainty with regard to if Zn^{2+} ions are released into the culture medium and then transferred to the cell, or if the ZnO NPs are endocytosed and release the ions thereafter. Based on the results of their study, the authors concluded that the toxicity of ZnO NPs is linked to cell uptake and subsequent release of Zn^{2+} ions into the cytoplasm, particularly in organelles such as lysosomes with lower pH values.

Guo et al. [45] highlighted the molecular mechanisms involved in calcium homeostasis mediated by plasma membrane calcium ATPase (PMCA) by studying the cytotoxicity of ZnO NPs on rat retinal ganglion cells (RGC). After verifying, through MTT assay, the toxicity of high-concentration ZnO NPs toward RGC-5 cells, the authors chose three different concentrations (2.5, 5, and 10 µg/mL) for subsequent experiments. Through the study in the expression of PMCA2, cell membrane transport proteins responsible for the ejection of Ca^{2+} ions from the cytosol, they hypothesized the possible Ca^{2+}-mediated signaling pathway, involved in the regulation of PMCA2 in the RGC-5 damage process caused by ZnO NPs. This mechanism hypothesized that ZnO NPs inhibit the activity of Ca^{2+} ATPase, increasing the levels of intracellular calcium ions and destroying intracellular calcium homeostasis, which in turn induces an overgeneration of ROS. The destruction of calcium homeostasis and the increase of ROS influence each other, leading to decreased expression of the PMCA2 gene and protein levels, thus initiating the apoptosis/necrosis mechanism of RGC-5 cells. The decrease in PMCA2 and protein levels was evidenced by the results of the quantitative polymerase chain reaction (Q-PCR) and enzyme-linked immunosorbent assay (ELISA) tests, which showed a decrease dependent on the ZnO concentration. The molecular mechanisms involved were also studied thanks to the help of real-time cell electronic sensing systems.

As noted above, the aerodigestive tract is considered to be particularly exposed to contact with NPs. In this regard, Moratin and co-workers [46] conducted a study comparing the cytotoxicity of malignant and non-malignant cell lines. They used human head and neck squamous cell carcinoma (SCCHN) derived from FaDu cells, chosen as a representative model of the mucosa of the upper aerodigestive tract, whereas they used human mesenchymal bone marrow stem cells (BMSCs) as non-malignant representatives. Cells were incubated at concentrations between 4 and 20 µg/mL for periods ranging from 1 to 48 h. The authors performed both the MTT assay and flow cytometry, in addition to fluorescence-activated cell sorting analysis (FACS), to improve the validity of the results. Both tests showed a reduction in cell viability, dependent on the ZnO NP concentration and exposure time. The mechanisms of apoptosis and necrosis appeared to be both responsible in the same way for cell death. Comparing the effects on the two cell lines, the applied doses of 5, 10, and 15 µg/mL were non-cytotoxic for the BMSCs, while the same concentrations diminished the cell viability of the FaDu cells, demonstrating the diversity of the effect on malignant and non-malignant cells. However, the comet assay revealed that, at low concentrations of 5 µg/mL, there was already significant DNA damage, even for non-malignant cells. In light of these results, the authors suggested a more critical and careful approach to the use of ZnO NPs in anticancer care.

After being absorbed at the respiratory, cutaneous, and gastro-intestinal levels, NPs can reach the blood and then migrate to different organs and systems, such as kidney, muscles, spleen, liver, and brain. When NPs come to the kidneys, they can impair metabolic functions and glomerular filtration; however, few studies are present on the toxicity of ZnO NPs on kidneys. A recent study by Reshna and Mohanan [47] focused on the in vitro toxicity of ZnO NPs on human embryonic kidney 293 (HEK 293) cells. The results showed a strongly concentration-dependent effect. From a morphological point of view, the transmission electron microscopy (TEM) analyses reported low changes at low concentrations, while, at 75 µg/mL ZnO NP concentration, the effects after 24 h of treatment were evident. To better consider the cytotoxic effects of ZnO NPs, the authors performed two independent studies: the MTT assay and the neutral red uptake assay (NR). The results showed a dose- and time-dependent toxicity. In the MTT assay, a net decrease in vitality was found at 25 µg/mL at each exposure time. The ROS concentration was measured, considered as the first mechanism of toxicity. Furthermore, changes were found in the actin distribution of HEK 293, depending on the dose of ZnO NPs used. Since actin filament is one of the critical elements in the cell division mechanism, such alterations in actin distribution can result in mitotic aberrations, leading to genomic instability. Changes were found in mitochondrial membrane potential, and lysosomal activity and the percentage of apoptotic cells were measured. Finally, through acridine orange staining (AO), autophagy (cell death type two) was determined, which is an important mechanism for the maintenance of cellular homeostasis, through the removal of damaged organelles, pathogenic organisms such as viruses and bacteria, etc. In addition, the appearance of some nuclear constrictions at high concentrations of ZnO NPs indicated dysfunctions in normal cell activity, due to DNA damage, leading to cell death by carcinogenesis.

In conclusion, from the results obtained in the aforementioned studies, it is possible to draw a synthetic scheme, reported in Figure 3, describing the mechanisms of interaction of ZnO NPs with the cell and the main causes of toxicity, explored further later.

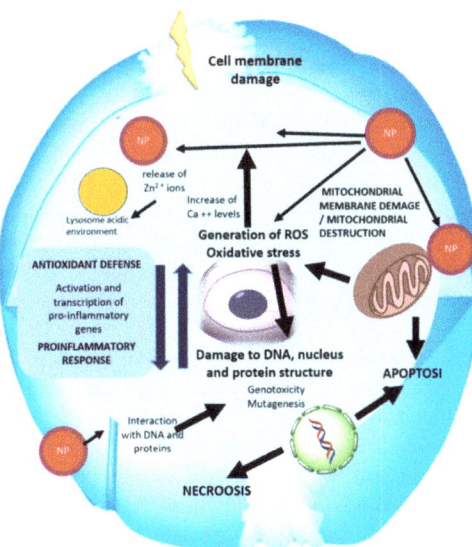

Figure 3. ZnO nanoparticle toxicity pathways mapped against a stylized cell.

2.2. Other Type of ZnO Nanostructures

In addition to the ZnO NPs, other hierarchical nanostructures acquired considerable interest in the biomedical field, thanks to their optic, optoelectronic, antibacterial, and detection sensitivity properties, as well as their selectivity with respect to particular cell lines, and the increase in cell proliferation and differentiation, which make them potential candidates for a new non-invasive approach for medical treatment [48–51]. The starting point, in order to open the way for future employment in the biomedical field of these NStr, is to understand how their morphological characteristics and physicochemical properties influence their toxicity and interaction with biological systems.

Paino et al. [52] investigated the cytotoxicity of flower-like nanostructures on Henrietta Lacks tumor cells (HeLa) and non-cancerous human fibroblast L929 cells, focusing on the effects of apoptosis and necrosis, ROS production, and cellular uptake. Cell viability tests were performed by incubating different forms of NFls for 24 h and at concentrations 0.1, 1, and 10 µg/mL, grown using a hydrothermal method at different times (4, 2, and 0.5 h). In particular, the NFls had rods of length between 1.7 and 2.3 µm and average diameters of about 250 nm. The results showed elevated cytotoxicity effects for HeLa cells, while the effects on non-carcinogenic cells were not statistically significant, showing that these nanostructures could be used for anticancer therapies without causing serious damage to healthy cells (in this case, fibroblasts). The morphological effects of NFls were also studied; the key parameter in determining differences in morphology was synthesis time. The internalization of NFls by HeLa induced cellular mortality by promoting oxidative-stress-dependent pathways, with increased intracellular ROS levels leading to necrosis.

Muller and co-workers [53] showed the effect of toxicity of ZnO NWs on human monocyte macrophages (HMMs) in cultures at similar concentration of $ZnCl_2$, demonstrating that the release of Zn^{2+} ions is one of the main processes involved in toxicity. The NWs were synthesized by electrodeposition and had thicknesses of about 120–320 nm and lengths from 2 to 10 µm, depending on the duration of the electrodeposition process. Cytotoxicity was investigated by NR assay, measuring the accumulation of neutral red dye in the lysosomes of live cells. ZnO NWs with high aspect ratio in a $ZnCl_2$ solution were incubated with the cells for 24 h at concentrations of 10, 20, and 40 µg/mL, showing similar toxicity, although only the concentration of 20 µg/mL showed statistically significant values. Confocal microscopy (CM) on cells confirmed an increase in the level of intracellular Zn^{2+} concentration before cell death. To better investigate the dissolution of the ZnO NWs, inductively coupled plasma mass spectroscopy analyses (ICP-MS) were performed in fluids at different pH values. They simulated a lysosomal acidic environment, as in the case of simulated body fluid-5 (SBF-5), and an environment mimicking the extracellular pH, and they recorded rapid dissolution in the first case compared to the second, demonstrating that dissolution firstly occurred inside the cells. Bright-field transmission electron microscopy (BF-TEM) showed a rapid uptake of the ZnO NWs. The HMM cells were incubated with 50 µg/mL ZnO NWs for 1 h; they showed a large phagocytosis of extensive aggregates of NWs. In conclusion, cell death presented features typical of apoptosis processes, such as condensation of chromatin and mitochondrial pyknosis, and of necrosis processes, such as plasma membrane rupture and leaching of cytoplasmic contents. The authors concluded that the ZnO NWs could be good candidates for drug-targeting, allowing modulation and control of the dissolution rate and delivery.

Gopikrishnan et al. [54] epitaxially grew ZnO NRs, with lengths of 50–60 nm and diameters of about 20–25 nm, using a hydrothermal method. They then evaluated their biocompatibility by analyzing their interaction with rat lung epithelial cells (LE). In particular, intracellular ROS levels were measured by studying the temporal kinetics of ROS production of LE treated with 2.5, 5, and 10 µg/mL ZnO NRs. After exposure, no increase in oxidative stress or lipid peroxidation was observed in the cells exposed, even at the highest periods of time and concentration levels. The MTT cell viability test showed independence of the viability of the LE cells relative to concentration and exposure time, always above 95%. These results, according to the authors, were due to the low concentration of released Zn^{2+}

ions. Therefore, the hypothesis of existence of a threshold limit value for the concentration of Zn^{2+} that induces toxicity, a value never reached in their experiments, was established.

A study by Ahmed et al. [55] highlighted the mechanisms of apoptosis and oxidative stress in human alveolar adenocarcinoma cells (A549) caused by ZnO NRs. The high level of antioxidant enzymes superoxide dismutase (SOD) and catalase (CAT) suggested that oxidative stress was one of the main mechanisms of toxicity. The results of the atomic absorption spectrometry confirmed the release of Zn^{2+} ions, showing that a concentration of 10 μg/mL Zn^{2+} was released for cultures with 100 μg/mL ZnO NR concentration. However, this concentration of Zn^{2+} proved to be not particularly cytotoxic for the A549 cells, a result that was consistent with previous studies that showed that these concentrations of Zn^{2+} are not sufficiently high to cause cytotoxic effects in human cells, unless there is a contact between the particles and the cells. The emergence of apoptotic processes was demonstrated by the fact that ZnO NRs upregulated the cell-cycle checkpoint protein p53, a transcription factor that regulates the cell cycle and can initiate apoptotic processes, and pro-apoptotic Bax protein, while downregulating proteins antiapoptotic survivin and Bcl-2. Furthermore, ZnO NRs induced the activity of caspase 3 and caspase 9, enzymes that play a fundamental role in the phases of cell apoptosis. All these results suggested that ZnO NRs induced apoptosis and oxidative stress in the A549 cells via p53, survivin, Bax, Bcl-2, and caspase 3 pathways.

Wang et al. [56] analyzed the biological effect of an array of densely packed and vertically aligned ZnO NWs on three types of excitable cells, the NG108-15 cancerous neuronal cell line, the HL-1 cardiac muscle cell line, and neonatal rat cardiomyocytes. MTT assays showed a statistically significant inhibitory effect by ZnO NWs on mitochondrial activity after one day of culture, especially on NG108-15 and HL-1 cells, compared to gold, glass, and polystyrene substrates. The NG108-15 cells, HL-1 cells, and cardiomyocytes had diameters of about 10–100, 20, and 13 μm, respectively, while the thickness of the NWs was about 300 nm. Every single cell was completely covered by the NWs. The inhibitory effect could be due to the penetration of the cell membrane by the NWs or the lack of adhesion of the cells to the substrate. In the first case, the penetration of the NWs into the membrane would be strongly influenced by their diameter; instead, in the second case, the engraftment failure could be due to the topography of the array, in particular the density and spacing of NWs, which can lead to an insufficiency in flatness of the surface required for cell adhesion. Another factor of toxicity could be the release of intracellular Zn^{2+} ions in the acid environment of lysosomes. This hypothesis is not, however, among the most probable because the NWs are fixed to a substrate and, therefore, the process of phagocytosis could be difficult. Another interesting aspect that emerged from this study is that primary cardiomyocytes seem to better tolerate the inhibitory effect of NWs. This result was consistent with previous studies on NPs that showed a selectivity to cytotoxicity on rapidly dividing cells compared to primary cells. The authors concluded that the biocompatibility of ZnO NWs can be raised, but it is difficult to do it in densely packed arrays.

Papavlassopoulos et al. [57] tested the biocompatibility of ZnO TPs on human dermal fibroblasts (NHDF) by highlighting the influence of cell culture conditions and material properties on cytotoxicity. They found that the toxicity of TPs was significantly lower than that of spherical NPs. Furthermore, the morphology of ZnO TPs influenced cellular toxicity in contrast to surface charges modified by UV light illumination or O_2 treatment and material age. Finally they observed that the direct contact of the material with the cells had greater toxicity than the transwell culture models that caused only an indirect effect through the released of zinc ions.

3. Toxicity Studies on ZnO Nanostructures In Vivo

In the previous paragraphs, the effect of the ZnO NStr on different cell lines in vitro was described. Here, we focus on the studies that were carried out in vivo to evaluate the interaction with organs and apparatus. Figure 4 describes the main routes taken by ZnO NStr, starting from absorption, up to their distribution and accumulation or expulsion.

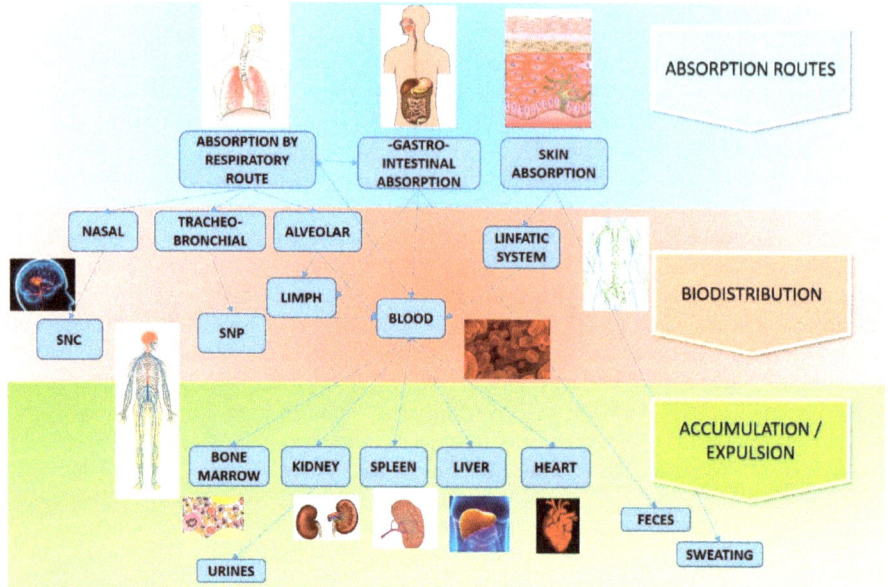

Figure 4. ZnO nanostructure (NStr) interaction mechanisms with the organism (SNC: central nervous system; SNP: peripheral nervous system).

Before starting with the description of recent in vivo studies, it is necessary to make a series of considerations in order to have a more conscious and focused approach for the analysis of the results obtained, as listed below.

- Most of the experiments were carried out on laboratory animals;
- In most cases, the doses were administered at one time and the concentration was significantly higher than the actual exposure conditions;
- There was no analysis of the long-term effects on the organism;
- There was no long-term study evaluating the effects due to exposure to small systemic concentrations.

Therefore, further analyses are required to have a comprehensive view of the effects of the ZnO NStr, looking for long-term effects and small exposure doses. However the results of the studies examined in this section provide a useful starting point for the assessment of risks associated with exposure to these nanomaterials.

Tian et al. [58] investigated the effects of neurotoxicity induced by ZnO NPs on differently aged mice, by studying the interaction between age and exposure to nanoparticles. According to the life cycle of CS7BL\6J mice, mice aged six months have a psychological age comparable to that of a 30-year-old man, while mice of 18 months can be compared to a man of 56 years; in both cases, we refer to healthy specimens. Firstly, the authors showed that ZnO NPs induced a systemic inflammatory response in both categories of mice, but with more severe effects in older mice, with a synergistic effect between the age of mice and exposure to NPs, with increased production of proinflammatory cytokines IL-1 and IL-6 in the blood. These data indicated that older individuals exhibited more severe inflammatory disorders during exposure with ZnO NPs. The neurotoxic effects were studied by intraperitoneal injection of 5.6 mg/kg ZnO NPs. Also, in this case, there was an increase in proinflammatory cytokines in the brain, with the same synergistic effect between age and exposure to NPs. In addition, significant increases in SOD and glutathione peroxidase (GSH-Px) concentration levels and increased malondialdehyde (MDA) concentration were observed, indicating oxidative stress conditions, especially in older individuals. The authors also analyzed the neurocognitive functions of mice. Data showed that long-term memory and passive avoidance ability were impaired following exposure to NPs, particularly in older mice. However, no significant changes in motor activity and in the exploratory behavior of mice were recorded. Instead, damage to spatial cognition was found, suggesting a link with the potential of the hippocampus, strongly linked to cognitive learning and memory skills. These dysfunctions are probably related to systemic inflammation of the central nervous system (CNS), which was further investigated by analyzing the levels of hippocampal proteins CREB and P-CREB, which decrease in age in a quantity-dependent manner. The authors stated the importance of the results obtained, although the doses were administered at one time and with high concentrations, with NPs of a single size. It is, therefore, essential to carry out further studies analyzing the effects of NP size and to evaluate chronic exposure at low concentrations.

Ansar et al. [59] examined the effects of hesperidin (HSP), 100 mg/kg body weight (bwt), on ZnO NPs during oral administration of 600 mg/kg bwt ZnO NPs in rats. The effects of neurotoxicity induced by NPs were evidenced by the increase in inflammatory markers, including TNF-α and proinflammatory interleukins. Furthermore, increases in C-reactive protein (CRP), CAT, GSH-Px, and glutathione (GSH) were recorded in the brains of rats, linked to the oxidative stress response. The administration of bioflavonoids such as hesperidin may play a protective role, inhibiting the induction of antioxidant enzymes and improving the ZnO NP-induced neurotoxicity. In fact, the results indicated a significant decrease in the levels of inflammatory cytokines in the blood of rats.

Liu et al. [60] studied the in vivo effects of the ZnO NPs on neuronal factors and on the neuroendocrine cells of the ovaries. For the study, concentrations of 25, 50, and 100 mg/kg (diet) ZnO NPs were used to treat pubertal hens. It was found that, at concentrations of 50 and 100 mg/kg, the ovarian organic index slightly decreased. Furthermore, the data indicated that the concentrations of essential elements in the ovaries, such as Zn, Fe, K, Ca, and Mn, increased, especially following exposure to the highest ZnO NP concentrations. The data showed that the increase in the concentrations of these elements was related to the levels in the genetic and protein expression of Neural Cell Adhesion Molecule 1 (NCAM1), Doublecortin (DCX), Roundabout Guidance Receptor 1 (ROBO1), Choline O-Acetyltransferase (CHAT), and neurofilament heavy (NF-H). The authors used quantitative transcriptomics (RNA-seq) to determine the effects of ZnO NPs on the gene expression of ovarian samples. It was found that 222 genes were modified by the treatment with ZnO NPs at 100 mg/kg, and, of these genes, 32 were related to neuronal factors (including those mentioned above) that are very important for organ development. To clarify the still unclear biological effect exerted by the ZnO NPs, or by the Zn^{2+} ion release, the authors used $ZnSO_4$ to compare these effects. They concluded that, in their study, both the ZnO NPs and the Zn^{2+} ions exerted their action on the biological system, since the ZnO NPs produced both effects similar to $ZnSO_4$ and specific effects, such as those on the regulation of neuronal factors in protein and gene expression.

Regarding the cytotoxic effects exerted by the ZnO NStr on the reproductive system, Han et al. [61] investigated the effects of ZnO NPs in vitro and on male mice. They studied cytotoxic effects in vitro on Leydig cells (LCs) and Sterol cells (SCs), and in vivo, via injection of a single dose on CD1 mice. LCs and SCs are two cell lines essential for the development of the gonads and for spermatogenesis; LCs play a fundamental role in the synthesis of steroidal testosterone, in sperm maturation, and in sexual functions, while SCs are located in the seminiferous tubules of the testes and provide nourishment, as well as structural and morphological support for germs during spermatogenesis. The results showed toxicity following the internalization of cell lines with ZnO NPs, manifested with apoptotic phenomena related to DNA damage and loss of mitochondrial membrane potential induced by ROS increase. In the in vivo tests, the authors observed significant reductions in the thickness of the seminiferous epithelium and in the diameter of the seminiferous tubules, in mice treated with a single injection of 5 mg/kg ZnO NPs. Furthermore, a statistically significant percentage of sperm showed morphological alterations such as double head, small head, double tail, etc. 49 days after treatment with ZnO NPs, with possible consequences on the fertility of mice.

Another organ in which the nanoparticles tend to accumulate is the kidney, causing toxicity on the cells and compromising important vital factors. Xiao et al. [62] focused on the toxic effects of ZnO NPs in vitro on podocytes and in vivo on rats. Variations of 10, 50, and 100 µg/mL were used to perform in vitro studies on podocytes, which showed induction of apoptosis by increasing intracellular ROS generation, as also confirmed by an experiment in which cells treated with N-mercaptopropionyl-glycine, known an ROS scavenger, showed decreased levels of apoptosis following exposure with NPs. The MTT assay revealed that the viability of the podocytes decreased in a dose- and time-dependent manner; in particular, a concentration of 100 µg/mL ZnO NPs caused a dramatic reduction in cellular activity. In in vivo acute toxicity studies, adult male Wistar rats were treated with 3 mg/(kg·day) ZnO NPs for five days. Decreases in important vital factors such as body weight and kidney index of rats were recorded, which suggested a potential toxicity of ZnO NPs on the kidney. Furthermore, the data showed a significant reduction in CAT and SOD levels, indicating an evident disturbance of the antioxidant functions, a result consistent with in vitro experiments. Finally, the loss of important proteins such as nephrine, a fundamental protein for the correct functioning of the renal filtration barrier and a structural component of the podocyte filtration barrier, was diagnosed. The latter aspect suggests to the authors that the ZnO NPs can interfere in the process of protein synthesis.

Concerning the genotoxic effects on different organs, Bollu et al. [63] assessed the effects of in vivo genotoxicity on Swiss Albino mice subjected to a dose ranging from 0.5 to 6 mg/kg of rod-shaped ZnO NPs of approximately 18 nm, administered orally for seven consecutive days. Their results showed no genotoxicity and no toxicity to the liver, heart, kidney, or spleen. In particular, the micronucleus assay was performed, a test to verify the formation of micronuclei during cell division processes and to indicate the presence of genotoxicity and chromosomal instability. The results of these tests showed the same percentages in the number of polychromatic erythrocytes in all the involved groups and compared to the control, indicating a non-dose-dependent effect. The chromosome aberration assay also demonstrated a non-significant increase in chromosomal aberration and the absence of chromosomal damage. Also, in this study, no percentage changes in the mitotic index were found, suggesting no incidence on cell proliferation. The alkaline comet assay reported no DNA damage caused by the ZnO NRs; in fact, there were no significant changes in the length of the comets. The results obtained are inconsistent with those of other research groups. The authors attribute these differences to the following possible motivations:

(1) The incidence of the shape and size of the particles; in fact, other studies reported that spherical and smaller nanoparticles are more likely to be taken up;
(2) The use, in this study, of small doses, comparable to those used in clinical procedures, which were much lower than those generally used in literature;
(3) The difference in conditions between in vitro and in vivo studies. The authors stressed the importance of the results obtained, but also the importance of carrying out further studies considering different routes of exposure, such as dermis, inhalation, etc.

4. New Approaches to Synthetize Safe ZnO Nanostructures for Biomedical Applications and Cancer Therapy

Numerous efforts are being made to synthesize biocompatible and safe ZnO nanostructures, suitable for use in the biomedical field. In this regard, Lewiński and his team [64] used a new organometallic self-supporting approach to synthesize "safety by design" ligand-coated ZnO nanocrystals (NCs). ZnO NCs of high quality and with size down to a quantum regime (<7 nm) were coated with densely packed 2-(2-methoxyethoxy) acetic ligands (MEAA), to obtain ZnO–MEAA NCs with average core size and hydrodynamic diameter of 4–5 nm and 12 nm, respectively. The characteristics of the nanocrystal–ligand interface, which gave protection to the core through an impermeable shell and a well-passivated surface, strongly influenced the physiochemical properties and biocompatibility of these nanostructures. In fact, in vitro cytotoxicity studies on normal human fetal lung fibroblast cells (MRC-5) and human lung cancer cells (A549), performed with MTT assay, showed low toxicity compared to structures of the same size synthesized with traditional methods, such as wet chemistry. In particular, even at the highest concentration tested of 25 µg/mL, the effects of toxicity were lower than the data in the literature about particles of the same size, despite using cell lines considered among the most sensitive. In addition, the ROS generation tests and the Zn^{2+} ion concentration reported relatively low values, indicating that the organometallic procedure conferred a good waterproof protection through the organic ligand shell, which inhibited the loss of Zn^{2+} ions by the core, improving surface stability. The authors conclude that this method can open new frontiers for the design of new, safe ZnO-based materials for biomedical applications.

Chun et al. [65] prepared zinc aminoclays (ZnACs) with functionalized primary amines ((–CH_2) $3NH_2$) via a sol–gel reaction, and studied their in vitro toxicity on HeLa cells and in vivo toxicity in zebrafish embryos. The purpose of their study was to compare the ZnACs with $ZnCl_2$ and $Zn(NO_3)_2$ salts and with ZnO NPs. In vitro studies on HeLa showed greater toxicity of ZnACs, probably caused by their greater bioavailability and uptake, as well as their positively charged hydrophilia caused by the production of ROS, especially in the case of ZnACs in their form of cationic nanoparticles. For in vivo toxicity analyses, the authors studied the duration of embryonic development at hatching in zebrafish exposed to ZnACs and ZnO NPs for 72 h. In both cases, a dose-dependent inhibition of embryo hatching was found. However, the ZnO NPs proved to be more toxic, probably due to their aggregation characteristics, colloidal behavior, and smaller hydrodynamic dimensions. However, the ZnACs reported toxicity effects on zebrafish embryos at the highest concentrations of 50 and 100 µg/mL.

ZnO nanostructures are proving very promising in drug delivery for the treatment of tumors, exploiting the selective effect of toxicity of ZnO particles toward the diseased cells, minimizing the impact on healthy cells. Zeng et al. [66] studied a lymphatic targeting drug delivery system for the treatment of lymphatic metastatic tumors, using lipid-coated ZnO NPs (LZnO-NPs). They synthesized core–shell nanoparticles (30 nm) loaded with 6-mercaptopurine (6-MP) using a water-in-oil (W/O) microemulsion. The MTT assay demonstrated the high selectivity of LZnO-NPs to cancer cells. In addition to the acid-sensitive behavior, an effective internalization of the particles in the cancer cells was enabled, with a rapid release of the drug in the cytoplasm and ZnO decomposition in the acid environment of the lysosomes. These results were also demonstrated by the acid sensitivity release experiment which indicated a prolonged drug retention time in the blood circulation (pH 7.4) and a rapid release in the lysosomes when the particles are internalized by the cells. The measurement of ROS levels showed a non-significant increase in primary lymphocytes due to their antioxidant capacity, which does not occur in cancerous cells where there is significant ROS accumulation. In vivo tests on Sprague-Dawley rats confirmed the higher biocompatibility of LZnO-NPs, compared to non-coated ZnO NPs; the red blood cell (RBC) tests showed that the RBCs did not aggregate in the presence of LZnO-NPs and there was no blood hemolysis, unlike the ZnO NP test. Biochemical parameters in the liver showed reversible hepatotoxicity in the case of LZnO-NPs, with parameters returning to control values, whereas hepatotoxicity was non-reversible in the case of ZnO-NPs. Histopathological analyses showed no significant lesions in the organs analyzed in the case of LZnO-NPs, while, in the case of ZnO-NPs, they showed mild–moderate inflammation in the intestine, kidneys, and lungs; LZnO-NPs only caused slight congestion in the spleen during the first hours of administration.

A new approach to breast cancer treatment was proposed by Vimala and his group [67]. They exploited the synergistic effect between chemo-photothermal targeted therapy and a multifunctional drug delivery system, developed through biosynthesis of polyethylene glycol (PEG)-coated ZnO nanosheets modified with folic acid (FA) after aminic functionalization (FA–PEG–ZnO NS), loaded with doxorubicin (DOX). The best results were found in the case of combined therapy, compared to that which exploited only the photothermal effect or only chemotherapy. The cancer cells in fact showed a good uptake and an effective internalization of DOX–FA–PEG–ZnO NS; in addition, under near-infrared irradiation (NIR), the maximum toxicity toward the breast cancer cells was found with respect to other cells and to the control. In vivo toxicity to mice was also tested, with results confirming the biocompatibility of the particles; a slight toxicity was observed for the liver linked to ROS production, while histopathological and morphological analyses on kidneys, lungs, brain, heart, and testes did not show abnormalities for these organs. Biocompatibility was also tested by injecting DOX–FA–PEG–ZnO NS through the tail vein, and the post-injured mice showed no pathology, and hematology markers did not show significant alterations.

5. Influence of the Chemical and Physical Properties of the ZnO Nanostructures on Toxicity

A key question regards the main mechanisms of toxicity induced by ZnO NStr, trying to understand the incidence of chemo-physical and morphological properties, such as size, shape, surface area, surface charge, and surface functionalization, as well as distribution, concentration, and aggregation phenomena. Reported studies showed that the main causes of cytotoxicity include the production of ROS (with consequent oxidative stress and lipid peroxidation), zinc ion release, the breakdown of the cell membrane, the impairment of mitochondrial functions, and DNA damage [40–42,46]. The results on the release of LDH confirmed that cellular rupture is among the main causes of toxicity, even if the results of MMT tests suggest that the mitochondrial functions are even more compromised [44]. The ZnO NStr also induce the production of immunoregulatory cytokines, which, on the one hand, can stimulate a defense response, and, on the other, they can cause long-term undesirable effects [41,58]. Other cytotoxicity mechanisms involve calcium homeostasis processes, as the ZnO NPs inhibit the activity of Ca^{2+} ATPase [45]. Furthermore, alterations in the expression values of some genes and protein levels were found to trigger apoptosis/necrosis mechanisms leading to cell death. Even alterations in cell division processes can lead to genomic instability [45,55].

With regard to the sensitivity of the different cell lines, considerable differences were observed. Among PBMC cells, the lymphocytes proved to be the most resistant cells, while the monocytes were among the most sensitive [40]. Moreover, within the lymphocytes, there were differences between native lymphocytes and memory lymphocytes, with proliferation-dependent toxicity levels. The rapidly dividing cells were more susceptible to the toxicity of the ZnO particles; this selectivity of the ZnO nanostructures makes them interesting in future perspectives for cancer treatment [41]. To confirm this, it was shown that the cytotoxic effects of ZnO are different depending on whether malignant and non-malignant cell lines are studied; the former are in fact more affected by the toxic effects of the particles [46,52]. Considering the different contact routes and the biodistribution of nanoparticles, the upper aerodigestive tract is considered one of the regions most affected by exposure to nanoparticles; in particular, the respiratory apparatus cells are among the first to come into contact with the ZnO NStr, which can in fact be easily inhaled [42,43]. Kidney cells also appear to be compromised in terms of metabolic and filtration functions.

The concentration of nanostructures is another crucial parameter for the determination of their toxicity, and it was shown to be concentration- and time-dependent [40]. Cell viability, in fact, decreases with increasing concentration and incubation time [43,44,46]. However, some other studies supported that the mechanism of association is maximum in the first hours of interaction, before stabilizing or, in some cases, reducing, possibly due to exocytosis phenomena [42]. Many studies highlighted the possible existence of a maximum threshold value for the concentration of ZnO NStr that does not compromise cell viability and, beyond which, the effects of toxicity increase as a function of the increase in concentration [43,54]. For the ZnO NPs, this value is around 5–10 µg/mL [43].

Figure 5 shows the vitality values for different cell lines as a function of ZnO concentration and considering 24 h of exposure; the values were extrapolated from the results of some of the studies described in the previous paragraphs. The trends obtained are purely qualitative and refer to extremely heterogeneous data that were affected by the variability of the experimental methodology, the different culture conditions, the density of cells used, and numerous other factors that make the comparison between the data not easy to interpret. However, useful general considerations can be made allowing a global overview of the results. In particular, in Figure 5a, the cellular vitality values normalized with respect to the initial cell density are reported in the ordinate, and the ZnO concentration is reported in the abscissa, expressed as molarity. The analyzed data are summarized in Table 1, where the value of the initial cell density, the type of culture plate, the type of vitality test, and the type and dimensions of nanostructure are indicated for each experiment. Observing the trends, we can appreciate the previous observations relating to the resistance of the different cell lines, as well as the influence of the concentration and the type of nanostructure examined. Figure 5b shows an enlargement of the ZnO concentration range, between 0 and 0.1 mM, i.e., from 0 to about 8 µg/mL, within which all the cell lines considered, with the exception of podocytes (which have limit values of lower concentration), show viability values above 70%, regardless of the type of nanostructure.

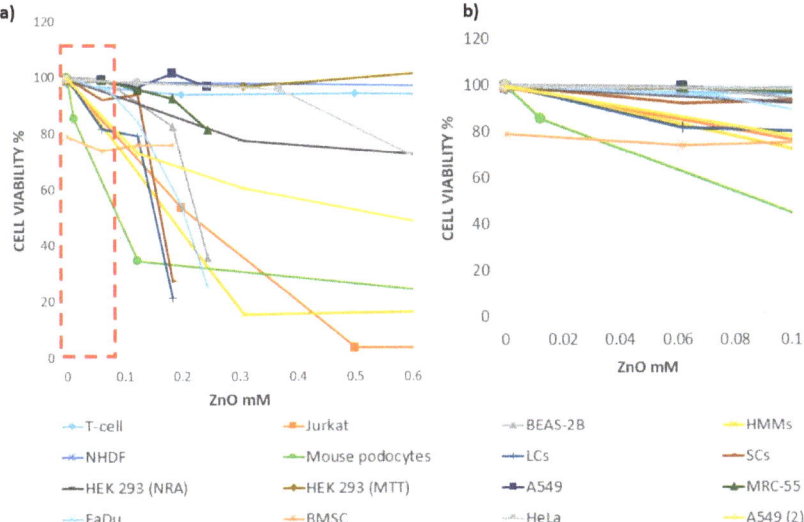

Figure 5. (**a**) Overall elaboration from published data about cell viability vs. ZnO concentration, for different cell lines and different types of nanostructures; (**b**) zoom-in of the red dashed area in (**a**), highlighting the ZnO concentration range where cell viability is preserved and is relatively "safe".

Relative to the influence of the size, a correlation was found between the production of ROS and the nanostructure size, with cytotoxicity inversely proportional to the size of the particles, whereby the smallest particles presented the highest levels of ROS concentration [40,42]. In addition, small particles are more likely to be involved in engrafting phenomena and subsequent phagocytosis. On the other hand, the nanostructures shape affects the dissolution rate. Solubility at different pH values modulates the release of Zn^{2+} ions; in particular, the release of ions in acidic culture environments, mimicking the lysosomal one, presents much higher values than those obtained in environments with a neutral pH [44,53]. Nanostructures of different shapes have different cytotoxic effects. Small and spherical nanoparticles exhibit the highest levels of ROS concentration; moreover, the greater association of the ZnO spherical nanoparticles makes them more suitable for anticancer and drug delivery treatments [42]. The ZnO NPs can in fact be designed to combine with antibodies or small molecules, peptides, or proteins associated with tumors and be destined for drug delivery applications. The ZnO NFls present different toxicity to cancer cells than healthy cells, with levels in the apoptotic indicators much higher in diseased cells, characteristics that make them suitable for anticancer applications [52]. The ZnO NWs present high dissolution values and have a tendency to aggregate; moreover, like the ZnO NPs, they manifest a rapid uptake and can be phagocytized, initiating apoptotic and necrotic processes [53,54]. They are also among the potential candidates for drug-targeting applications [53]. ZnO NRs have lower levels of toxicity with higher threshold values than other nanostructures; however, at sufficiently high concentrations, they can initiate apoptotic processes and lead to oxidative stress [54,55].

Table 1. Description of the systems analyzed in the graphic reconstruction of Figure 5. MTT, 3-(4,5 -dimethylthiazol-2-yl)-2,5-diphenyltetrazolium bromide assay; L/D, live/dead viability/cytotoxicity assay; WST, Cell Counting Kit 8 assay; NR, neutral red assay; TB, trypan blue assay.

Ref	C0	Well Type	Cell Line	ZnO NStr Type	ZnO NStr Dimensions	Cell Viability Assay
[41]	1×10^5 cells/well	96-well plates	T-cell	NPs	4–20 nm	L/D
[41]	5×10^4 cells/well	96-well plates	Jurkat	NPs	4–20 nm	L/D
[42]	5×10^4 cells/well	12-well culture dish	BEAS-2B	NPs	~10 nm	WST
[53]	-	96-well plates	HMMs	NWs	120 nm × 2–5 μm	NR
[44]	5×10^4 cells/cm^2	Flat 96-well plates	NHDF	TRPs	~37 nm	MTT
[62]	1×10^4 cells/mL in each well	96-well plates	Mouse podocytes	NPs	20–80 nm	MTT
[61]	1×10^4 cells/well	96-well plates	LCs	NPs	70 nm	MTT
[61]	1×10^4 cells/well	96-well plates	SCs	NPs		MTT
[47]	1×10^4 cells/well	96-well plates	HEK 293	NPs	25–40 nm	NR
[64]	1×10^4 cells/well	96-well plates	A549	NCs	4.7 ± 0.8 nm	MTT
[64]	1×10^4 cells/well	96-well plates	MRC-5			MTT
[46]	1×10^5 cells/well	96-well round-bottom plates	FaDu	NPs	20 nm	MTT
[46]	1×10^5 cells/well	96-well round-bottom plates	BMSC	NPs		TB
[65]	10^4 cells/mL	96-well plates	HeLa	NPs	~50 nm	WST
[55]	1×10^4 cells well	96-well plates	A549 (2)	NRs	diameter ≈ 52 nm	MTT

Despite the great importance of the results obtained in vitro, the in vivo approach is very different and more complex, due to the increased number of variables involved. The absence of an official protocol, the diversity in the selected concentrations, which are often administered in a single dose and with much higher values than the clinical ones, the great complexity of the biological interactions, and the variability of the physiological boundary conditions make the interpretation of the results obtained in tests on animal models an extremely complex process [58,61–63]. According to the in vitro results, increases in SOD, MDA, and proinflammatory cytokine production were also measured in in vivo tests [58]. Neurotoxicity studies showed evidence of long-term memory impairment and spatial cognition, probably caused by systemic inflammation of the central nervous system, as evidenced by the measured levels of hippocampal proteins and the increase in inflammatory markers [58]. Studies on neuroendocrine cells highlighted alterations in the concentration of essential elements in the ovaries, linked to levels in gene and protein expression [60]. The reproductive system of male mice presented morphological changes in the sperm, including reduction of the thickness of the seminiferous epithelium and the diameter of the seminiferous tubules [61]. Harmful effects caused by exposure to ZnO NPs were also found in the kidneys, with reduction of important vital factors such as kidney index and degradation of the filtering functions [61]. Other organs subjected to the toxicity of the nanoparticles are the liver, spleen, pancreas, lungs, and brain. However, studies on

ZnO rod-shaped nanoparticles reported non-significant effects of toxicity in the liver, kidney, spleen, and heart, in addition to the absence of genotoxicity, confirming some results of in vitro studies that showed the lower toxicity of this type of nanostructure [63].

Some new research lines focused on the development of Zn–ZnO nanostructures, engineered with particular functional groups, core–shell coated, hybrid organic–inorganic, often obtained through the use of biosynthesis methods, with the aim of increasing their biocompatibility or enhancing some properties and strengthening their use in the biomedical field and in oncology. The results in vitro and in vivo showed the greatest biocompatibility of these constructs, which have lower levels of toxicity compared to the traditional ZnO NStr [64–67].

6. ZnO–Polymeric Hybrid Electrospun Nanomaterials

6.1. Tissue-Engineering Applications

Tissue engineering (TE) aims to design new materials suitable for replacing/repairing damaged organs/tissues, thus avoiding a number of transplants or complex and expensive interventions [68]. The use of particular nanostructures can improve the biocompatibility of these materials, as well as recreate environments that mimic the native extracellular matrix, providing the mechanical, structural, and chemical–physical characteristics suitable to promote the biological interactions necessary to guarantee the compatibility of the scaffolds [69]. Among the metal oxides, ZnO is one of the most investigated for tissue-engineering applications, thanks to its antibacterial properties and to its role in promoting cell growth, proliferation, and differentiation [70]. These properties were experimentally studied for pure ZnO nanostructures [71] and in combination with composite materials, mainly polymers and ceramics [72,73], in order to realize 3D scaffolds manufactured using additive manufacturing techniques. ZnO NStr were tested to analyze their role in osteointegration processes. In this context, the selected nanomaterial must possess biomechanical properties to confer the restoration of the tissues, promote their growth, induce the formation of new bone, and guarantee the vascularization [71]. Park et al. [74] studied the in vitro, on MC3T3-E1 osteoblast, and in vivo osteointegration processes on two different ZnO-based nanostructures, i.e., a thin film and an array of nanoflowers, both grown on silicon substrates by pulsed laser deposition, and, in the second case, following photolithography. The promotion of osteointegration processes, as well as the antibacterial properties of ZnO nanostructures, makes them promising materials even in periodontal applications, such as dental materials and implants [75]. Memarzadeh and co-workers investigated a mixed coating of ZnO NPs and nanohydroxyapatite (NHA) on a glass substrate for the promotion of the growth of osteoblasts and antibacterial functions for possible applications in orthopedic and dental implants.

An essential requirement for TE is the biocompatibility of nanostructures in terms of cell viability and adhesion, as well as within the mechanisms involved in cell growth, proliferation, and differentiation processes. Ciofani and his collaborators [76] tested these properties on an array of ZnO NWs using two electrically excitable cell lines, namely, the PC12 cell line, which was suitable for modeling neuronal cells, and the H9C2 line, which was instead suitable for modeling muscle cells. With regard to differentiation, PC12 showed a well-developed neurite network, while H9C2 showed poor development of regular myotubes, presenting disordered dispositions, an aspect that was attributed to the different mechanical interaction between the cells and the substrate. Neuronal-type cells prefer a rather rigid substrate, such as the one used in this case; on the contrary, the muscle cells need a softer substrate for the correct fusion in myotubes.

Very recently Errico et al. [77] experienced a reversible myogenic–differentiation switching, effecting the functionalization of a glass substrate by means of a dense ZnO NWs array. The results of these studies suggested that, depending on the type of cell line, the ZnO NWs arrays can promote or inhibit cell differentiation.

The combination of inorganic components and organic matrices such as biopolymers improve the physicochemical properties, enabling them to satisfy the delicate balance between structure, biocompatibility, and stability [78]. Moreover, since the toxicity of ZnO nanostructures is concentration-dependent, the use of a methodology that incorporates the nanostructures within a matrix reduces their toxicity and increases the time required for their degradation.

Among the numerous synthesis techniques, electrospinning proved a promising approach for the production of hybrid polymeric nanoconstructs [79]. The basic set-up consists of a needle nozzle, a high-voltage power supply, a container for spinning fluid, and an electrode collector [80]. The electrospinning process depends on a number of parameters that can critically affect fiber formation and structure [81]. The study of interrelation between such parameters and nanofiber properties are considered very crucial for cell–scaffold interactions and cell growth. Depending on the cell type, specific electrospinning parameters have to be chosen for the achievement of optimal pore dimension, porosity, fiber diameter, and orientation [82].

Regarding the solution parameters, it is necessary that the concentration of the starting solution varies within a useful range. In fact, for concentrations below a minimum, a set of fibers and grains are obtained (beads), while, beyond a maximum concentration, it is impossible to maintain a constant flow at the level of the needle tip. The molecular weight influences instead the electrical and rheological properties and, therefore, the morphological characteristics of the fibers. In fact, the molecular weight reflects the number of bonds between the polymer chains in solution [29]. The selection of a desirable solvent is fundamental for the optimization of electrospinning. In fact, the surface tension depends substantially on the type of solvent and on the difference in solubility, while the viscosity of the solution and the high relative humidity can contribute to the formation of pores in the electrospun fibers [83,84]. Recent studies focused on the use of less toxic solvents for electrospinning, although the choice of these solvents requires an accurate optimization process [85].

Process parameters such as applied voltage, tip-to collector distance, type of collector, and the electric field have effects on the jet impact speed. The electrospinning process starts at a threshold voltage able to induce the polarization of the solution; the speed with which the syringe is fed influences the speed of the jet and the solvent evaporation process. Generally, low feed rates are more desirable since the solvent has more time to evaporate, whereas too high fluxes result in the formation of granular fibers due to the inadequacy of the achieved evaporation level [86,87]. A minimum distance between the tip and the collector is needed to allow the solvent to evaporate before it reaches the collector, thus avoiding the formation of unwanted granules in the final structure; moreover, the needle tip-to-collector distance has a considerable influence on the nanofiber diameter and the nanoweb collection zone [88].

Numerous biopolymers were used in combination with ZnO for tissue-engineering applications; among them, poly(ε-caprolactone) (PCL) has numerous advantages such as biocompatibility and biodegradability [89], and it is approved by the Food and Drug Administration (FDA) and used in clinical applications [90].

With regard to antibacterial and tissue regeneration properties, Bottino et al. [91] tested the potential application for periodontal regeneration of PCL/ZnO NPs and a PCL gel/ZnO NP electrospun scaffold. In particular, they studied the antibacterial properties of these composite materials against two known periodontal pathogenic bacteria: *Porphyromonas gingivalis* (Pg) and *Fusobacterium nucleatum* (Fn). They used 0.5, 15, and 30 wt.% ZnO, and they observed that, upon increasing ZnO content, antibacterial properties improved, but cell viability worsened, an aspect tested on human dental stem cells (hDPSCs). A good compromise was achieved using a 15 wt.% ZnO scaffold. An inhibition of bacterial activity was found, especially toward Fn; the PCL gel structure instead influenced the antimicrobial activity toward Pg. In particular, the presence of the gel changed the behavior of the scaffold from hydrophobic to hydrophilic, increasing the wettability of the fabric. The PCL gel also showed better mechanical properties in terms of tensile strength, Young's modulus, and elongation at break.

An important property of the PCL/ZnO hybrid material lies in its electrical conductivity. Sezer and his group [92] explored this aspect for the regeneration of neuronal tissue. They used zero-valent zinc NPs at different concentrations (5, 10.15, and 20 wt.%) in solution together with PCL, making the material through electrospinning; they tested linear electrical conductivity, mechanical properties, the proliferation of U87 glioblastoma cells, and the toxicity on fibroblasts. The morphological properties of the fibers changed according to the Zn content, but a direct correlation between fiber diameter and Zn content was not identified. Regarding the mechanical properties, all the samples containing Zn had better values than the fibers containing only PCL. Electrical conductivity is a fundamental parameter for cells capable of being electrically stimulated, such as neuronal tissue cells; the results showed that the conductivity of fibers with 5 wt.% and 10 wt.% Zn was approximately equal to that of the nervous tissue. The authors emphasize the positivity of the results and conclude that further studies are needed to investigate the effect of the catalytic activity of Zn NPs on neuronal cells.

Augustine [93] and his group tested a PCL/ZnO composite scaffold focusing on the angiogenic mechanisms induced by commercial ZnO NPs loaded on an electrospun scaffold intended for TE. They used PCL with different percentages of ZnO NPs ranging from 0.5 to 4 wt.%. The scaffolds with 1 and 2 wt.% showed the best behavior both in cell proliferation tests in vitro, conducted on human dermal fibroblasts (HDFa), and in the test of chorioallantoic egg membrane (CAM), which showed the formation of blood vessels following the insertion of the scaffold. For this reason, the scaffold with 1 wt.% ZnO NPs was selected for the next subcutaneous implantation in guinea pigs for five days. During this test, the formation of mature blood vessels and a branched capillary network was demonstrated, as well as the migration of fibroblasts from the walls toward the inside of the scaffold. Furthermore, a circular arrangement of red blood cells was observed, indicating the beginning of an angiogenic process. Finally, the Western blot test showed that the main cause of angiogenesis activation was linked to the presence of small percentages of ZnO NPs that stimulated the production of proangiogenic factors, expressed by fibroblast growth factor-2 (FGF2) and vascular endothelial growth factor (VEGF) proteins.

Another interesting polymer for TE applications, thanks to its piezoelectric properties, is polyvinylidene fluoride (PVDF). Li and co-workers [94] analyzed PVDF and ZnO as potential bone TE materials. In their study, PVDF scaffolds doped with ZnO NPs (ZnO/PVDF) were prepared by electrospinning increasing ZnO concentrations and the ratio of the β-phase PVDF. The results showed an improvement of the elasticity modulus, elongation at break, and maximum load; in addition, piezoelectrically excited scaffolds exhibited much greater osteoblast density than control and compared to unexcited scaffolds, indicating that the piezoelectric ZnO/PVDF scaffolds can promote osteoblast proliferation through piezoelectricity.

While the PVDF needs to be mechanically stretched to form the piezoelectric crystalline phase (beta phase), the co-polymer polyvinylidene fluoride–trifluoroethylene (PVDF–TrFE) instead possesses a permanent piezoelectric nature and does not need mechanical stretching before the poling. Its intrinsic electrical properties were studied for the enhancement of neuritis extension [95], to manipulate the fibroblast cellular behavior and proliferation. Augustine et al. [96] recently studied the biocompatibility of (PVDF–TrFE)/ZnO nanocomposite scaffolds in terms of cell adhesion and formation of blood vessels. The polymer was loaded with different percentages of ZnO, from 1 to 4 wt. %. In vitro cell cultures were made using human mesenchymal stem cells (hMSCs) and human umbilical cord endothelial cells. In vivo tests were performed on the Wistar rats, in which the formation of a highly branched capillary network of blood vessels was found. Moreover, in this study, the piezoelectric properties of the scaffold were taken into consideration, as a stimulating cause of a better cellular response. In fact, the electrical potential generated by the piezoelectric scaffold can convert the mechanical energy generated by the cellular environment into electrical signals that increase the cellular response. This aspect was highlighted by the Fourier-transform infrared spectroscopy (FTIR) analysis, which indicated a relative abundance of the electro-active β-phase of the nanocomposite material, compared to the net scaffold.

In addition to the polymers already considered, numerous other biocompatible polymers were used, in combination with ZnO, in electrospinning processes aimed at producing materials for tissue regeneration. Amna et al. [97] produced a spider web using polyurethane (PU) and ZnO NPs. The particular bimodal structure, which alternated fibers with a larger diameter and very thin fibers similar to spider webs, was probably generated by the ionization of the polymeric solution in the presence of ZnO NPs. Furthermore, the presence of ZnO increased the overall crystallinity of the polymer. The same group [98] made one-dimensional ZnO-doped TiO_2 by electrospinning using a colloidal gel composed of zinc nitrate, titanium isopropoxide, and polyvinyl acetate (PVA), which was subsequently annealed at 600 °C for 2 h. They used a standard Cell Counting Kit 8 (CCK-8) assay to study the effects of the material on adhesion, proliferation, and growth of C2C12 myoblasts. Balen et al. [36] produced a nanostructured composite of poly(methyl methacrylate) (PMMA) and ZnO NPs at concentrations of 0, 3, 5, 10, and 15 wt.%, using two different techniques: casting, to obtain a film, and electrospinning, to make a fibrous construct. They then studied the structural, thermal, and optical properties and the biocompatibility of the two materials. The results showed, in the case of fibrous material, that the ZnO content reduced the diameter of the fibers and the number of bids, as well as exhibiting greater hydrophobicity. For both categories, the ZnO improved the optical properties of the composite, with an intense absorption around 320 nm and a high luminescence in the ultraviolet (UV) region. Biological tests showed a better behavior of the material made with electrospinning, thanks to the greater surface area and its greater affinity and morphological similarity with the extracellular matrix; the fibroblast cells indeed showed greater vitality, further improved by the ZnO NP content. Percentages of ZnO higher than 1 wt.% increased the biocompatibility of the material; however, at 15 wt.% concentration, the cell proliferation was inhibited, due to the cytotoxic effect exerted by the ZnO NPs. Table 2 summarizes the main results obtained from the studies discussed in this paragraph, related to tissue-engineering applications.

6.2. Wound-Healing Applications

A hotspot application in the medical field is certainly represented by "wound healing" following trauma, surgical operations, implants, etc. A good wound dressing must be able to ensure an environment suitable for wound healing and must, therefore, guarantee a sufficient level of moisture, allow the exchange of gas, prevent the occurrence of infections caused by microorganisms, allow the removal of exudates, and minimize the scar formation. In addition, it must be non-toxic, non-allergenic, easily removable, and biocompatible [99]. Recently, the use of inorganic antimicrobials, including metal nanoparticles, gained considerable interest due to their broad antimicrobial spectrum, and their lower tendency to develop bacterial resistance [100,101]

The antibacterial and catalytic properties of ZnO and its biocompatibility make it an excellent candidate for wound-healing applications as it promotes regeneration and re-epithelialization of tissues and prevents scar formation [102].

Recent studies proposed various solutions that combine ZnO with different kinds of dressing in the form of gelatin/ointments [103], hydrogel [104–106], or electrospinning mats [107], made mainly with synthetic polymers or natural polymers or even a mix. Figure 6 shows a comparison between fibrous tissues manufactured by electrospinning, hydrogels, and electrospun gelatinous fibers.

Focusing on electrospinning, Shalumon and his research team [108] fabricated a sodium alginate (SA)/poly(vinyl alcohol) (PVA)/ZnO NP fibrous mat and studied the antibacterial properties toward *Staphylococcus aureus* (*S. aureus*) and *Escherichia coli* (*E. coli*) bacteria and the biocompatibility on L929 cells, proposing such a material for wound-healing applications. In addition, they analyzed the influence of ZnO on fiber properties such as viscosity, conductivity, and thermal stability. The results obtained showed that the insertion of the ZnO NPs had a slight effect on the viscosity and a more marked influence on the conductivity, which increased with the increase in ZnO content. The blend of SA/PVA was more stable to thermal decomposition when compared with the individual polymers, while thermal stability did not seem to be particularly enhanced by the presence of nanoparticles. Antibacterial studies demonstrated that the mats showed an inhibition zone in both bacteria for all ZnO concentrations, directly proportional to the ZnO concentration. Cytotoxicity studies indicated that fibers with 0.5 and 1 wt.% ZnO concentrations are less toxic, while cell viability decreased as the ZnO concentration increased. The authors concluded that there was a need to find an optimal concentration with the least toxicity while providing maximum antibacterial activity.

Table 2. Main results of recent studies on ZnO-based nanomaterials and electrospun ZnO-polymeric hybrid nanomaterials for tissue-engineering applications.

Type of System	Ref	Description of the System	ZnO Concentration	Cell Line/Bacteria	In Vivo Experiments	Main Results
ZnO NStr/ZnO array for experimental purposes	[74]	ZnO NFIs arrays on Si substrate	Zinc nitrate solution 25 mM	MC3T3-E1 osteoblast culture	Implantation on calvarial bone defects of Sprague Dawley rats	Formation of lamellipodia and filopodia
	[75]	ZnO NWs arrays incubated with a collagen solution		PC12 and H9C2	–	Adhesion, proliferation, and differentiation of two different electrically excitable mammalian cell lines
	[77]	ZnO NWs arrays on a glass substrate		Mesoangioblasts	–	- Reversibly locked differentiation - No cell damage - Differentiation capabilities completely recovered upon cell removal from the nanowire substrate and re-plating on standard culture glass
ZnO/PCL electrospun scaffold	[90]	PCL+ZnO NPs	0.5–6 wt.%	HDFa	Implantation in guinea pigs	- Proangiogenic properties of ZnO/PCL fibers - Increase in the formation of mature blood vessels and highly branched capillary network
	[91]	PCL and PCL/gelatin + ZnO NPs	0, 5, 15, 30 wt.%	Pg, Fn, hDPSCs, AllCells LLC, Alameda, CA.	–	- Potential application in periodontal regeneration - Good antibacterial properties
	[92]	PCL matrix + zero-valent Zn NPs	5, 10, 15, 20 wt%	Neuroglioblastoma cells, human primary fibroblasts	–	Small concentrations of Zn NPs promoted neuronal cell proliferation with relative non-toxicity for fibroblasts
ZnO-polymeric (other polymers) electrospun implantable scaffold	[97]	ZnO-PU scaffold	5 wt%	mouse fibroblast	–	Fibroblast viability, adhesion, and proliferation
	[95]	(PVDF–TrFE) + ZnO NP scaffold	0, 0.5, 1, 2, 4 wt.%	Red blood cells, White blood cells, platelet, hMSCs), HUVECs	Subcutaneous implantation in Wistar rats	- Tissue regeneration due to the piezoelectric properties of the composite components - Biocompatibility of the system in vitro - Angiogenic properties in vivo
	[94]	β-phase PVDF + ZnO NPs	0.5, 1, 2 mg/mL	Human osteoblasts, S. aureus, methicillin-resistant S. aureus, E. coli.	–	- Improvement of the elongation modulus at break and load stress - Greater osteoblast density and antibacterial properties of the piezoelectrically excited scaffold
	[98]	1D ZnO-doped TiO$_2$ fabricated using colloidal gel	1 and 10 µg/mL of ZnO/TiO$_2$	C2C12 myoblast cells	–	Beneficial effect on the adhesion, proliferation, and growth of myoblasts
	[96]	PMMA + ZnO NPs fibers and films	0, 1, 3, 5, 10, 15 wt.%.	Fibroblast cells (L929)	–	- Good proliferation of fibroblast cells - Thermal stability - Luminescence with emission in the near-UV range

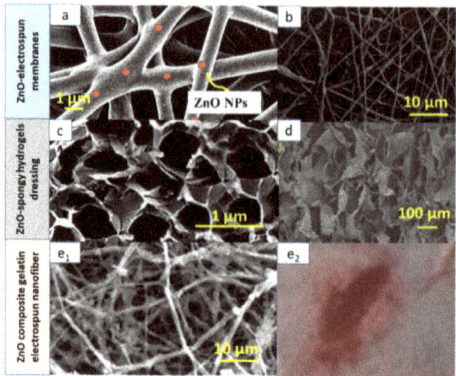

Figure 6. Wound-healing solutions. (**a**) Higher-magnification SEM micrograph of poly(ε-caprolactone) (PCL) membrane containing 1 wt.% ZnO nanoparticles, (**b**) SEM image of poly(3-hydroxybutyrate-co-3-hydroxy-valerate) (PHBV) reinforced with cellulose nanocrystal (CNC)–ZnO at weight loadings of 5%. (**c**) SEM image of keratin–chitosan-ZnO nanocomposite hydrogel. (**d**) SEM image of surface of chitosan (CS)–Ag/ZnO-1.0 (sponge immersed in 1.0 mg/mL of Ag/ZnO solution); (**e1**) SEM image of cefazolin-loaded zinc-oxide nanoparticle composite gelatin nanofiber, and (**e2**) dorsal skin region of rat embedded with the same nanofiber wound dressing.

Augustine and his collaborators [109] demonstrated the in vivo cell proliferations and wound-healing properties of an electrospun PCL/ZnO NP membrane. ZnO nanoparticle-embedded membranes did not show any significant sign of inflammation. A PCL membrane with 1 wt.% ZnO was implanted subcutaneously in a guinea pig's dorsal cervical defect. The scaffold did not show any significant sign of inflammation and, compared to pristine one, had better proliferation, cellular vitality, adhesion, and growth of fibroblasts, which migrated from the subcutaneous regions toward the skin, promoting wound healing with wound closure without scarring. The C-reactive protein test (CRP), measuring the concentration of a protein produced by the liver in response to an inflammation/infection, by means of pig blood agglutination tests, also demonstrated the good properties of the selected scaffold.

Abdalkarim et al. [110] produced electrospun nanofibrous membranes from cellulose nanocrystal–ZnO (CNC–ZnO) nanohybrids as reinforcing materials in biodegradable poly(3-hydroxybutyrate-co-3-hydroxy-valerate) (PHBV). The incorporation of CNC–ZnO nanocrystals improved the uniformity and reduced the diameter of the PHBV nanofibers. With regard to mechanical properties, an improvement in tensile strength and Young's modulus for nanofibrose membranes with 5.0 wt.% CNC–ZnO concentration was found. Furthermore, an increase in the initial decomposition temperature and the maximum decomposition temperature values was recorded. The nanofibrous membranes presented a positive effect on barrier properties and absorbency of simulated fresh blood. The 5.0 wt.% CNC–ZnO membrane showed the best antibacterial activity against *E. coli* and *S. aureus* bacteria. This nanocomposite hybrid material showed good results for potential use in antibacterial wound dressing.

Ahmed and his team [111] designed new chitosan/PVA/ZnO electrospun nanofibrous mats for diabetic wound healing. They demonstrated the antibacterial properties against *E. coli*, *Pseudomonas aeruginosa* (*P. aeruginosa*), *Bacillus subtilis* (*B. subtilis*), and *S. aureus*, which were better than those of fibers made with only chitosan/PVA; furthermore, the nanocomposite also had superior antioxidant properties. The authors also tested wound-healing skills in vivo on subcutaneous wounds in diabetes-induced rabbits (six months and weight of 0.8 to 1.3 kg). The results showed that chitosan/PVA/ZnO nanofibrous membranes resulted in accelerated wound healing. The mix between the biocompatibility and non-toxicity of PVA, the properties of chitosan (which promote a rapid contraction of wounds, and stimulate the proliferation of fibroblasts, the formation of collagen, and the deposition of hyaluronic acid in the vicinity of the wound), and the antibacterial and angiogenic properties of ZnO NPs made this material a good dressing for diabetic wounds. In conclusion, the authors stated that new studies to better understand the mechanism of action of this material, in addition to analyzing its genotoxicity, together with experiments on human subjects, will be necessary.

Rath et al. [112] combined the antimicrobial properties of ZnO NPs and cefazolin, a drug usually adopted for the treatment of post-operative wounds, exploiting both the fibrous morphology that can be obtained through electrospinning and the properties of gelatin, which is a bioavailable, economic polymer that presents good swelling and allows counteracting fluid losses due to exudation, improving wound healing. They manufactured cefazolin-loaded zinc-oxide nanoparticle composite gelatin nanofiber mats (both separately and in combination) for post-surgical operation wounds. Firstly, they determined the minimum inhibition concentration for cefazolin, ZnO NPs, and their mixture against *S. aureus*; then, they performed in vitro tests on the antibacterial properties and final in vivo experiments to evaluate the capacity of wound healing on Wistar rats. The results showed sustained drug release behavior and good antibacterial efficacy, especially for ZnO and cefazolin in a 1:1 weight ratio. From the in vivo tests, it was found that the hybrid material had more rapid and effective wound healing compared to the fibers loaded with drugs only or ZnO NPs only; moreover, the histological examinations revealed a greater cell adhesion, re-epithelialization, and production of collagen by the composite material.

Kantipudi et al. [103] used AgNPs and Ag-ZnO composite NPs (0.1 g NPs) formulated into gel using the Carbapol 934 as a base gel, and they tested their ability to wound healing in vivo on excision wound (4 cm length and 2 mm depth) in adult male Albino Wistar rats. The composite showed good wound healing ability from the early stages, and after 10 days the wound showed fibrosis, caused by rapid epithelialization of the skin, indicating maximum effectiveness of healing. The wounds treated with only Ag NPs did not exhibit fibrosis, probably due to the insufficient antibacterial capacity compared to the composite material. Finally, in the case of using a standard dermazine drug, the healing process appeared very slow.

Figure 7 depicts the in vivo test results described in References [109,112], while Table 3 summarizes the main results with regard to wound healing.

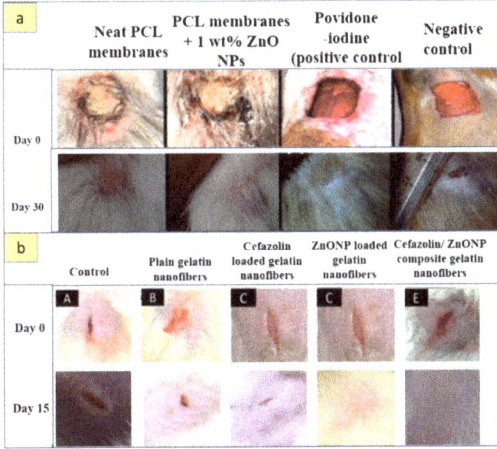

Figure 7. Results of different wound-healing dressing solutions in vivo. (**a**) Wound-healing activity of the membrane. The first column indicates neat PCL membranes, the second column indicates a PCL membrane incorporated with 1 wt.% ZnO NPs, the third column indicates povidone–iodine-treated wounds (positive controls), and the fourth column indicates negative controls. (**b**) Physical estimation of wound healing at various time intervals in the control (A), plain gelatin nanofibers (B), cefazolin-loaded gelatin nanofibers (C), ZnO NP-loaded gelatin nanofibers (D), and cefazolin/ZnO NP composite gelatin nanofibers (E) (adapted from [109], with permission from RSC, 2019, and from [112], with permission from Elsevier, 2019).

Table 3. Main results of recent studies on ZnO-based nanomaterials and electrospun ZnO–polymeric hybrid nanomaterials for wound-healing applications.

Type of System	Ref	Description of the System	ZnO Concentration	Cell Line/Bacteria	In Vivo Experiments	Main Results
Electrospun fibrous membranes	[105]	Sodium alginate/poly(vinyl alcohol) fibrous mat + ZnO NPs	0.5, 1, 2.5 wt.%	L929 fibroblasts cells, S. aureus, E. coli		- Fibers with 0.5 and 1% ZnO concentrations are less toxic - Inhibition for both the bacteria - Toxicity increase at the high ZnO concentration.
	[108]	PCL + ZnO NPs	1, 2, 4 wt.%		Membranes implanted subcutaneously in guinea pigs	- ZnO enhanced the cell adhesion, migration, and proliferation -No significant sign of inflammation - In vivo implant enhanced the wound healing without any scar formation
	[110]	Cellulose nanocrystal (CNC)–ZnO in poly(3-hydroxybutyrate-co-3-hydroxy-valerate)	CNC–ZnO suspension at 0, 3, 5, 10, 15 wt.%	E. coli and S. aureus		- Improvement in tensile strength and in Young's modulus - High thermal stability -Good antibacterial activity
	[111]	Chitosan/PVA/ZnO NP nanofibrous membranes		E. coli, P. aeruginosa, B. subtilis, S. aureus	Subcutaneous wounds in diabetes-induced rabbits	- High antibacterial and antioxidant potential - ZnO accelerated wound healing in vivo
	[104]	Ag/ZnO into chitosan sponge	Immersion in 0.1, 0.2, 0.5, and 1.0 mg/mL of Ag/ZnO and in 0.5 mg/mL of ZnO solution	S. aureus, E. coli, P. aeruginosa, human normal hepatocyte (L02)	BALB/c mice: wound with a length of 7 mm on the back	- Evaluation of the porosity, swelling, blood clotting, and in vitro antibacterial activity - Low toxicity in vitro - Enhanced wound healing, re-epithelialization, and collagen deposition in vivo
Spongy hydrogels	[105]	Hydrogels of heparinized PVA/chitosan/ZnO NPs		Mouse fibroblast cells (L-929), E. coli, S. aureus		- Heparin release rate decreased by adding ZnO NPs - Good antibacterial protection of wounds
	[106]	Porous keratin–chitosan/n-ZnO hydrogel	ZnO nanopowder 0, 0.5, 1 wt.%	fibroblasts cells (NIH 3T3), E. coli, S. aureus	Sprague-Dawley rats: skin wound of 1.5 cm^2 in the dorsum of the rat	- Biocompatibility in vitro. - Increased wound curing in vivo with quicker skin cell construction and collagen development
Gel and gelatin nanofibers or ointments	[112]	Cefazolin + ZnO NPs electrospun gelatin nanofiber mats	1:1 w/w combination of cefazolin and ZnO NPs (1–64 μg/mL)	In vitro release studies + antibacterial property for S. aureus	Wistar rats: 2-cm-long incision	- Therapeutic approaches for post-operative wound - Determination of minimum inhibitory concentration - Hybrid antibacterial nature of ZnO NPs and cefazolin - Accelerated wound healing
	[29]	AgNPs and Ag–ZnO NPs formulated into gel using Carbapol 934	0.1 g of NPs		Adult male albino Wistar rats: excision wound (4 cm length and 2 mm depth)	- Wound-healing properties of Ag–ZnO NPs in vivo - Rapid healing within 10 days when compared with pure AgNPs and standard drug, dermazin

6.3. Antimicrobial Materials

The tendency to use metal compounds, including the ZnO-based ones, inside polymer matrices allowed creating new multifunctional materials with antibacterial and antifungal properties [113] to be used for a wide range of sectors, including photocatalytic materials for the degradation/removal of polluting species [114,115], materials for water treatment/separation [116], antiseptic and antibacterial membranes for the biomedical sector, food packaging, special self-cleaning fabrics [117], super-hydrophobic and antibacterial surfaces, and many others [118]. The confinement/anchoring of the nanostructures inside or on the surface of the polymers allows reducing the toxicity, optimizing the useful active concentrations, and creating a synergic effect between the properties of the different phases of the composite material obtained [119]. The antibacterial properties of ZnO can also be used for food storage and preservation; among the various solutions, one of the most promising involves the creation of an active antibacterial food packaging in which the material in contact with food is able to modify its characteristics and the environment that surrounds it [120,121]. The incorporation of ZnO inside polymeric matrices allows obtaining an active food packaging able to provide the proper antibacterial properties and to increase the mechanical and thermal properties of the packaging [122]. Figure 8 summarizes the properties of these new antibacterial ZnO–polymeric materials, the main antibacterial action mechanisms, and applications in which these materials are intended.

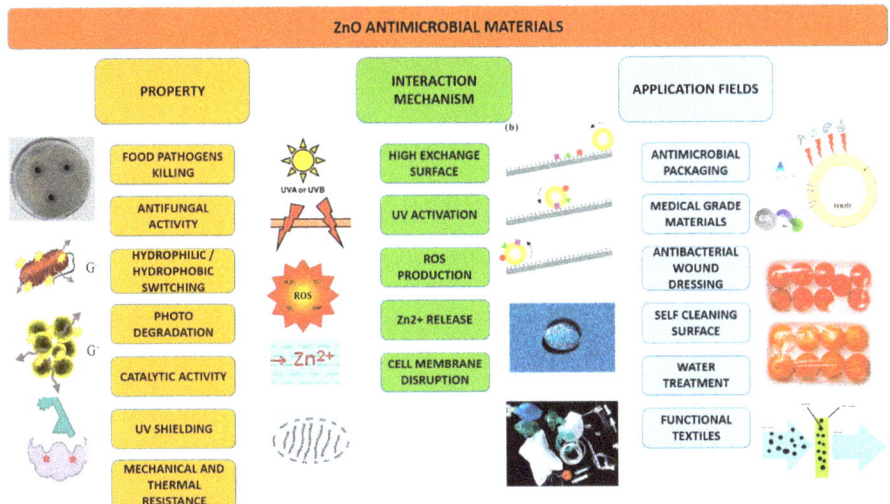

Figure 8. Properties, mechanisms of action, and applications of new ZnO-based antimicrobial materials.

Electrospinning proved to be an effective and promising technique for the construction of these new antibacterial tissues with multifunctional properties, as described in the examples below. Wang et al. [123] created hierarchical nanofibers of electrospun polyamide-6 (PA-6) subsequently subjected to atomic layer deposition (ALD) and a hydrothermal method for the deposition and growth of ZnO "water lily"- and "caterpillar"-like NRs. They then studied the antibacterial properties against *S. aureus* and found that the caterpillar-like NRs had better antibacterial activities, as indicated by the larger diameter of the inhibition zone; however, further studies are needed to understand the contributions of ALD cycles and the hydrothermal reaction period to the antibacterial properties.

The photocatalytic and optical properties of ZnO can be exploited to enhance the overall antibacterial effect. Prone and co-workers [124] recently developed mats with coaxial and uniaxial fibers of PCL and Zn-based NPs by electrospinning and studied their antibacterial properties toward *E. coli* and *S. aureus* under the action of UV-A light. They used different concentrations of ZnO NPs in the 9–25 wt.% range and selected this range because no significant inhibition of planktonic growth and biofilm bacteria was previously found at concentrations below 9%. During the electrospinning process, they studied the effect caused by the addition of ZnO NPs on the surface charge density of the jet and found that, as the concentration of ZnO increased, the stretching forces exerted under the action of the electric field increased, with a consequent reduction in diameter of the fibers. The Energy-dispersive X-ray spectroscopy (EDS) results demonstrated homogeneity in the distribution of NPs within the fibers, an important aspect to guarantee the uniformity of the antibacterial properties. Moreover, in the case of coaxial fibers, the NPs were mainly concentrated in the outer layer, due to the lower polarization of the jet's inner core, an advantageous aspect to increase the antibacterial surface extension; in the uniaxial fibers, the NPs were instead mainly confined inside. The authors also demonstrated that the presence of ZnO NPs reduced the hydrophobicity of the tissue compared to the use of pristine PCL fibers; moreover, the ZnO NPs facilitated the degradation of PCL, reducing its crystallinity. The turbidity test showed that the nanocomposite exerted an inhibitory action of the planktonic growth caused mainly by the release of Zn^{2+} ions and by the photocatalytic oxidation process. In fact, if the tissue was illuminated with UV-A for 15 min before the inoculation of the bacteria, there was an increase in the photocatalytic production of ROS by the ZnO NPs, especially in the case of coaxial fibers.

Anitha et al. [125] manufactured ZnO nanoparticle-embedded cellulose acetate (CA) fibrous membranes by electrospinning and tested their optical, antibacterial, and water-repellent properties. Also, in their work, the technique of electrospinning proved to be effective in avoiding the agglomeration of the particles and maximizing the active antibacterial surface. According to the results of other studies, the antibacterial action was stronger against *S. aureus* than toward *E. coli*, probably due to the different structural nature of the bacteria cell walls, which, in the case of *S. aureus*, is presented as a multilayer porous membrane of peptidoglycan and is, thus, more susceptible to intracellular transition of nanoparticles. However, antibacterial activity against *Klebsiella pneumoniae* (*K. pneumonia*) was not reported. With regard to the wettability tests, the results of the contact-angle measurements indicated that the properties of the CA passed from hydrophilic to hydrophobic due to the ZnO impregnation. The material was suitable for use as an antibacterial hydrophobic surface without the need for further surface treatments.

Kim et al. [126] developed, by electrospinning, polyurethane (PU) nanofibers coated with polydopamine (Pdopa) using a deep coating method and subsequently put them into a ZnO NP solution as a seed layer for the hydrothermal growth of ZnO NRs. The NR film obtained adhered firmly to the surface of the PU fibers, and the results showed excellent photocatalytic and antibacterial performances under the action of light-emitting diode (LED) devices with low UV intensity. The photocatalytic activity was investigated by monitoring the degradation of a blue methylene (MB) solution by measuring the absorbance via a UV–visible spectrophotometer. The authors speculated that this material, thanks in part to its high reusability and durability, may be suitable for developing antifungal photocatalytic membranes or for degrading organic pollutants and purifying wastewater.

Malwal and Gopinath [127] synthesized CuO–ZnO composite nanofibers using electrospinning and subsequent calcination for water treatment applications; they then measured their antibacterial properties, absorption kinetics, absorption isotherm, and diffusion characteristics. The combination of antibacterial and absorption properties made this material suitable for water treatment and purification processes.

Liu and co-workers [128] fabricated electrospun nanofibers starting from ethylcellulose/gelatin solutions containing various concentrations of ZnO NPs. The presence of ZnO as a filler allowed increasing the hydrophobicity of the tissue, the water stability, and the antibacterial action toward *E. coli* and *S. aureus*, especially after UV irradiation. The authors stated that, thanks to these properties, the material could potentially be used in food packaging. Table 4 offers a summary of these results.

Table 4. Main results of recent studies on ZnO-based nanomaterials and ZnO-polymeric composite nanomaterials for sustainability applications.

Type of System	Application	Ref	Description of the System	ZnO Concentration	Cell Line/Bacteria	Main Results
ZnO Coating	Antimicrobial activity against food pathogens	[120]	ZnO (ZnO nanoparticle suspension)-coated Polyvinyl chloride film	93.75 and 187.5 ug/cm^2	E. coli, S. aureus, fungal Aspergillus flavus and Penicillium citrinum	- Antimicrobial activities of Polyvinyl chloride-based films to inactivate food pathogens - Effective antibacterial activity for S. aureus - No antifungal activity
	Advanced functional textile	[127]	ZnO NP-coated polyvinylsilsesquioxane (PVSQ) composite	0, 0.3, 0.5, 1, 2, 3 g	E. coli and S. aureus	- Excellent UV shielding and stable superhydrophobic properties - Enhanced mechanical properties and thermal stability - Larger resistivity of the E. coli compared to the S. aureus
	Hydrophobic-bactericidal materials	[125]	ZnO NPs embedded on CA fibrous membrane	0.2 mol of zinc acetate dihydrate	Staphylococcus aureus, E. coli, Klebsiella pneumoniae, Citrobacter freundii	- Hydrophobic nature of the surface - Strong antibacterial activity
	Antibacterial application	[123]	PA-6 nanofiber modified with ZnO using ALD + hydrothermal reaction	100–150 cycles of ALD with ZnO seed layers (14.6 nm)	S. aureus	Efficient in suppression of bacteria survivorship
Electrospun nanocomposite membranes	Removal of biological/organic contaminants for water treatment and purification	[127]	CuO–ZnO-PVA nanofibers	50, 100, 150, 200, 250, 300, 350 ug/mL	E. coli and S. aureus	- Enhanced adsorption efficiency and antibacterial properties - Excellent adsorption capacity for congo red dye
	Photocatalysis and antimicrobial activity for organic pollutant degradation and waste water purification	[126]	Hierarchical ZnO NR deposited on PU nanofiber		E. coli	- High photocatalytic/antimicrobial activity at the low-intensity UV LED device with good reusability - Measure of the degradation of the methylene blue (MB) solution
	Antibacterial nanocomposite wound dressings	[124]	ZnO NP-PCL uniaxial or coaxial fiber structure	ZnO NPs 9, 12, 15 and 25 wt.% relative to PCL	E. coli, S. aureus	- Inhibition of planktonic and biofilm bacterial growth - Increased antibacterial properties for coaxial fibers and for exposure to UV-A light prior to bacteria inoculation
Gelatin composite films	Active shrimp packaging	[121]	ZnO NRs/clove essential oil incorporated into type B gelatin composite films	NR loading concentration 2% w/w of gelatin	Listeria monocytogenes and Salmonella typhimurium	- Film with low flexibility and high mechanical resistance- Oxygen and UV barrier property increased with ZnO NR incorporation - Composite films loaded with 50% clove essential oil and with ZnO NRs showed maximum antibacterial activity

7. Conclusions

The toxicity of Zno NStr strongly depends on their physical, chemical, and morphological (shape, size) properties. Toxicity is typically concentration- and time-dependent, and there is a threshold value below which the use of ZnO nanostructures does not appear to compromise cell viability. This value is lower for smaller, spherical, and higher-aspect-ratio ZnO NPs, while it increases for nanostructures such as ZnO NRs. In fact, as the nanostructures become smaller and more reactive, with a high surface-to-volume ratio, the cell uptake increases. Solubility at different pH and aggregation phenomena are other parameters that influence cytotoxicity. Among the main causes, the production of ROS, zinc ion release, breakdown of the cell membrane, impairment of mitochondrial functions, DNA damage, and the activation of apoptosis and necrosis processes were highlighted. The selectivity of ZnO NStr toward malignant and non-malignant cell lines makes them interesting for cancer therapy applications. The in vivo studies, although they are still limited, and although the administration of nanostructures is at higher concentrations than the clinical ones, confirmed the results obtained in vitro and showed that the most compromised organs are the kidneys, liver, spleen, pancreas, lungs, reproductive system, and the brain. In conclusion, it is necessary to carry out a careful study of the doses and times of administration of the nanostructures, as well as choosing the most suitable shape and size according to the target application, for an effective and safe use of these nanomaterials. Electrospinning is able to create macroscopic textile materials and coatings that inherit the properties of the constituent ZnO NStr. Clearly, the optimum in terms of concentration and type has to be determined vs. performance in terms of biological targets by means of rational design tools such as applied statistics and experiment design. Applications in wound healing and antibacterial barriers enabled by electrospinning promise to be particularly disruptive.

Author Contributions: The contributions of all the authors are equal.

Funding: This research received no external funding.

Conflicts of Interest: The authors declare no conflicts of interest.

References

1. Sousa, V.C.; Segadães, A.M. Combustion synthesized ZnO powders for varistor ceramics. *Int. J. Inorg. Mater.* **2002**, *1*, 235–241. [CrossRef]
2. Lin, Y.; Chen, Y. Effect of ZnO nanoparticles doped graphene on static and dynamic mechanical properties of natural rubber composites. *Compos. Part A Appl. Sci. Manuf.* **2015**, *70*, 35–44. [CrossRef]
3. Kandavelu, V.; Kastien, H. Photocatalytic degradation of isothiazolin-3-ones in water and emulsion paints containing nanocrystalline TiO2 and ZnO catalysts. *Appl. Catal. B Environ.* **2004**, *48*, 101–111. [CrossRef]
4. Yebra, D.M.; Kiil, S. Dissolution rate measurements of sea water soluble pigments for antifouling paints: ZnO. *Prog. Org. Coat.* **2006**, *56*, 327–337. [CrossRef]
5. Shi, L.E.; Li, Z.H. Synthesis, antibacterial activity, antibacterial mechanism and food applications of ZnO nanoparticles: A review. *Food Addit. Contam. Part A Chem. Anal. Control. Expo. Risk Assess.* **2014**, *31*, 173–186. [CrossRef]
6. Mu, L.; Sprando, R.L. Application of Nanotechnology in Cosmetics. *Pharm. Res.* **2010**, *27*, 1746–1749. [CrossRef]
7. Lewicka, Z.A.; Yu, W.W. Photochemical behavior of nanoscale TiO2 and ZnO sunscreen ingredients. *J. Photochem. Photobiol. A Chem.* **2010**, *263*, 24–33. [CrossRef]
8. Ozgur, Ü.; Hofstetter, D. ZnO devices and applications: A review of current status and future prospects. *Proc. IEEE* **2010**, *98*, 1255–1268. [CrossRef]
9. Wang, X.; Song, J. Nanowire and nanobelt arrays of zinc oxide from synthesis to properties and to novel device. *J. Mater. Chem.* **2007**, *17*, 711–720. [CrossRef]
10. Becheri, A.; Dürr, M. Synthesis and characterization of zinc oxide nanoparticles: Application to textiles as UV-absorbers. *J. Nanoparticle Res.* **2008**, *10*, 679–689. [CrossRef]

11. Hasnidawani, J.N.; Azlina, H.N. Synthesis of ZnO nanostructures using sol-gel method. *Procedia Chem.* **2016**, *19*, 211–216. [CrossRef]
12. Poornajar, M.; Marashi, P. Synthesis of ZnO nanorods via chemical bath deposition method: The effects of physicochemical factors. *Ceram. Int.* **2016**, *42*, 173–184. [CrossRef]
13. Solis-Pomara, F.; Jaramillo, A. Rapid synthesis and photocatalytic activity of ZnO nanowires obtained through microwave-assisted thermal decomposition. *Ceram. Int.* **2016**, *42*, 18045–18052. [CrossRef]
14. Ucer, K.B.; Pal, U. Synthesis and optical properties of ZnO nanostructures with different morphologies. *Opt. Mater. (Amst)* **2006**, *29*, 65–69.
15. Azam, A.; Ahmed, A.S. Antimicrobial activity of metal oxide nanoparticles against Gram-positive and Gram-negative bacteria: A comparative study. *Int. J. Nanomed.* **2012**, *7*, 6003–6009. [CrossRef] [PubMed]
16. Laurenti, M.; Cauda, V. ZnO Nanostructures for Tissue Engineering Applications. *Nanomaterials* **2017**, *7*, 374. [CrossRef] [PubMed]
17. Stubbs, N.; Lansdown, A.B.G. Zinc in wound healing: Theoretical, experimental, and clinical aspects. *Wound Repair Regen.* **2007**, *15*, 2–16.
18. Cai, X.; Luo, Y. PH-Sensitive ZnO Quantum Dots-Doxorubicin Nanoparticles for Lung Cancer Targeted Drug Delivery. *Acs Appl. Mater. Interfaces* **2016**, *8*, 22442–22450. [CrossRef] [PubMed]
19. Politi, J.; Rea, I. Versatile synthesis of ZnO nanowires for quantitative optical sensing of molecular biorecognition. *Sens. Actuators B Chem.* **2015**, *220*, 705–711. [CrossRef]
20. Zang, Z.; Tang, X. Enhanced fluorescence imaging performance of hydrophobic colloidal ZnO nanoparticles by a facile method. *J. Alloys Compd.* **2015**, *619*, 98–101. [CrossRef]
21. Ahmed, B.; Dwivedi, S. Mitochondrial and Chromosomal Damage Induced by Oxidative Stress in Zn^{2+} Ions, ZnO-Bulk and ZnO-NPs treated Allium cepa roots. *Sci. Rep.* **2017**, *7*, 1–14. [CrossRef]
22. Ahtzaz, S.; Nasir, M. A study on the effect of zinc oxide and zinc peroxide nanoparticles to enhance angiogenesis-pro-angiogenic grafts for tissue regeneration applications. *Mater. Des.* **2017**, *132*, 409–418. [CrossRef]
23. Zhang, R.; Huang, Q. ZnO nanostructures enhance the osteogenic capacity of SaOS-2 cells on acid-etched pure Ti. *Mater. Lett.* **2017**, *215*, 173–175. [CrossRef]
24. Parnia, F.; Yazdani, J. Overview of Nanoparticle Coating of Dental Implants for Enhanced Osseointegration and Antimicrobial Purposes. *J. Pharm. Pharm. Sci.* **2017**, *20*, 148–160. [CrossRef] [PubMed]
25. Wingett, D.; Louka, P. A role of ZnO nanoparticle electrostatic properties in cancer cell cytotoxicity. *Nanotechnol. Sci. Appl.* **2016**, *9*, 29–45. [CrossRef] [PubMed]
26. Sharma, B.; Malik, P. Biopolymer reinforced nanocomposites: A comprehensive review. *Mater. Today Commun.* **2018**, *16*, 353–363. [CrossRef]
27. Lin, R.; Hernandez, B.V. Metal organic framework based mixed matrix membranes: An overview on filler/polymer interfaces. *J. Mater. Chem. A* **2018**, *6*, 293–312. [CrossRef]
28. Hemamalini, T.; Rengaswami, V. Comprehensive review on electrospinning of starch polymer for biomedical applications. *Int. J. Biol. Macromol.* **2018**, *106*, 712–718. [CrossRef]
29. Haider, A.; Haider, S. A comprehensive review summarizing the effect of electrospinning parameters and potential applications of nanofibers in biomedical and biotechnology. *Arab. J. Chem.* **2018**, *11*, 1165–1188. [CrossRef]
30. Ding, J.; Zhang, J. Electrospun polymer biomaterials. *Prog. Polym. Sci.* **2019**, *90*, 1–34. [CrossRef]
31. Ponnamma, D.; Cabibihan, J.J. Synthesis, optimization and applications of ZnO/polymer nanocomposites. *Mater. Sci. Eng. C* **2019**, *98*, 1210–1240. [CrossRef] [PubMed]
32. Sun, B.; Li, X. Electrospun poly(vinylidene fluoride)-zinc oxide hierarchical composite fiber membrane as piezoelectric acoustoelectric nanogenerator. *J. Mater. Sci.* **2019**, *54*, 2754–2762. [CrossRef]
33. Pascariu, P.; Homocianu, M. Preparation of La doped ZnO ceramic nanostructures by electrospinning–calcination method: Effect of La^{3+} doping on optical and photocatalytic properties. *Appl. Surf. Sci.* **2019**, *476*, 16–27. [CrossRef]
34. Han, J.; Xiong, L. Bio-functional electrospun nanomaterials: From topology design to biological applications. *Prog. Polym. Sci.* **2019**, *91*, 1–28. [CrossRef]
35. Ginestra, P.; Ceretti, E. Electrospinning of Poly-caprolactone for Scaffold Manufacturing: Experimental Investigation on the Process Parameters Influence. *Procedia CIRP* **2016**, *49*, 8–13. [CrossRef]

36. Balen, R.; Vidotto, W. Structural, thermal, optical properties and cytotoxicity of PMMA/ZnO fibers and films: Potential application in tissue engineering. *Appl. Surf. Sci.* **2016**, *385*, 257–267. [CrossRef]
37. Aziz, A.; Tiwale, N. Core–Shell Electrospun Polycrystalline ZnO Nanofibers for Ultra-Sensitive NO2 Gas Sensing. *Acs Appl. Mater. Interfaces* **2018**, *10*, 43817–43823. [CrossRef]
38. Bafqi, M.S.S.; Bagherzadeh, R. Fabrication of composite PVDF-ZnO nanofiber mats by electrospinning for energy scavenging application with enhanced efficiency. *J. Polym. Res.* **2015**, *22*, 130. [CrossRef]
39. Hou, J.; Wu, Y. Toxic effects of different types of zinc oxide nanoparticles on algae, plants, invertebrates, vertebrates and microorganisms. *Chemosphere* **2018**, *193*, 852–860. [CrossRef]
40. Hanley, C.; Thurber, A. The influences of cell Type and ZnO nanoparticle size on immune cell cytotoxicity and cytokine induction. *Nanoscale Res. Lett.* **2009**, *4*, 1409–1420. [CrossRef]
41. Hanley, C.; Layne, J. Preferential killing of cancer cells and activated human T cells using ZnO nanoparticles. *Nanotechnology* **2008**, *19*, 29. [CrossRef] [PubMed]
42. Heng, B.C.; Zhao, X. Toxicity of zinc oxide (ZnO) nanoparticles on human bronchial epithelial cells (BEAS-2B) is accentuated by oxidative stress. *Food Chem. Toxicol.* **2010**, *48*, 1762–1766. [CrossRef] [PubMed]
43. Heng, B.C.; Zhao, X. Evaluation of the cytotoxic and inflammatory potential of differentially shaped zinc oxide nanoparticles. *Arch. Toxicol.* **2011**, *85*, 1517–1528. [CrossRef] [PubMed]
44. Wang, B.; Zhang, Y. Toxicity of ZnO Nanoparticles to Macrophages Due to Cell Uptake and Intracellular Release of Zinc Ions. *J. Nanosci. Nanotechnol.* **2014**, *14*, 5688–5696. [CrossRef] [PubMed]
45. Guo, D.; Bi, H. Zinc oxide nanoparticles decrease the expression and activity of plasma membrane calcium ATPase, disrupt the intracellular calcium homeostasis in rat retinal ganglion cells. *Int. J. Biochem. Cell Biol.* **2013**, *45*, 1849–1859. [CrossRef]
46. Moratin, H.; Scherzad, A. Toxicological Characterization of ZnO Nanoparticles in Malignant and Non-Malignant Cells. *Environ. Mol. Mutagenesis.* **2018**, *59*, 247–259. [CrossRef] [PubMed]
47. Reshma, V.G.; Mohanan, P.V. Cellular interactions of zinc oxide nanoparticles with human embryonic kidney (HEK 293) cells. *Colloids Surf. B Biointerfaces* **2017**, *157*, 182–190.
48. Okyay, T.O.; Bala, R.K. Antibacterial properties and mechanisms of toxicity of sonochemically grown ZnO nanorods. *Rsc Adv.* **2015**, *5*, 2568–2575. [CrossRef]
49. Singh, A.; Singh, S. ZnO nanowire-coated hydrophobic surfaces for various biomedical applications. *Bull. Mater. Sci.* **2018**, *41*, 94. [CrossRef]
50. Girigoswami, A.; Ramalakshm, M. ZnO Nanoflower petals mediated amyloid degradation-An in vitro electrokinetic potential approach. *Mater. Sci. Eng. C* **2019**, *101*, 169–178. [CrossRef]
51. Bahramian, R.; Eshghi, H. Influence of annealing temperature on morphological, optical and UV detection properties of ZnO nanowires grown by chemical bath deposition. *Mater. Des.* **2016**, *107*, 269–276. [CrossRef]
52. Paino, I.M.M.; Gonçalves, F.J. Zinc Oxide Flower-Like Nanostructures That Exhibit Enhanced Toxicology Effects in Cancer Cells. *Acs Appl. Mater. Interfaces* **2016**, *8*, 32699–32705. [CrossRef] [PubMed]
53. Müller, K.H.; Kulkarni, J. PH-dependent toxicity of high aspect ratio ZnO nanowires in macrophages due to intracellular dissolution. *Acs Nano* **2010**, *4*, 6767–6779. [CrossRef] [PubMed]
54. Gopikrishnan, R.; Zhang, K. Epitaxial growth of the Zinc Oxide nanorods, their characterization and in vitro biocompatibility studies. *J. Mater. Sci. Mater. Med.* **2011**, *22*, 2301–2309. [CrossRef] [PubMed]
55. Ahamed, M.; Akhtar, M.J. ZnO nanorod-induced apoptosis in human alveolar adenocarcinoma cells via p53, survivin and bax/bcl-2 pathways: Role of oxidative stress. *Nanomed. Nanotechnol. Biol. Med.* **2011**, *7*, 904–913. [CrossRef]
56. Wang, Y.; Wu, Y. Cytotoxicity of ZnO Nanowire Arrays on Excitable Cells. *Nanomaterials* **2017**, *7*, 80. [CrossRef] [PubMed]
57. Papavlassopoulos, H.; Mishra, Y.K. Toxicity of Functional Nano-Micro Zinc Oxide Tetrapods: Impact of Cell Culture Conditions, Cellular Age and Material Properties. *PLoS ONE* **2014**, *9*. [CrossRef]
58. Tian, L.; Lin, B. Neurotoxicity induced by zinc oxide nanoparticles: Age-related differences and interaction. *Sci. Rep.* **2015**, *5*, 1–12. [CrossRef]
59. Ansar, S.; Abudawood, M. Exposure to Zinc Oxide Nanoparticles Induces Neurotoxicity and Proinflammatory Response: Amelioration by Hesperidin. *Biol. Trace Elem. Res.* **2017**, *175*, 360–366. [CrossRef]
60. Liu, X.Q.; Zhang, H.F. Regulation of neuroendocrine cells and neuron factors in the ovary by zinc oxide nanoparticles. *Toxicol. Lett.* **2016**, *256*, 19–32. [CrossRef]

61. Han, Z.; Yan, Q. Cytotoxic effects of ZnO nanoparticles on mouse testicular cells. *Int. J. Nanomed.* **2016**, *11*, 5187–5203. [CrossRef] [PubMed]
62. Xiao, L.; Liu, C.; Chen, X.; Yang, Z. Zinc oxide nanoparticles induce renal toxicity through reactive oxygen species. *Food Chem. Toxicol.* **2016**, *90*, 76–83. [CrossRef] [PubMed]
63. Sravan Bollu, V.; Soren, G. Genotoxic and Histopathological Evaluation of Zinc Oxide Nanorods in Vivo in Swiss Albino Mice. *J. Evol. Med. Dent. Sci.* **2016**, *5*, 6186–6192. [CrossRef]
64. Pietkiewicz, M.W.; Tokarska, K. Safe-by-design' ligand coated-ZnO nanocrystals engineered by an organometallic approach: Unique physicochemical properties and low negative toxicological effect toward lung cells. *Chem. Eur. J.* **2018**, *24*, 4033–4042. [CrossRef] [PubMed]
65. Chun, H.S.; Park, D. Two zinc-aminoclays' in-vitro cytotoxicity assessment in HeLa cells and in-vivo embryotoxicity assay in zebrafish. *Ecotoxicol. Environ. Saf.* **2017**, *137*, 103–112. [CrossRef]
66. Zeng, H.; Zhang, Z. Lipid-coated ZnO nanoparticles as lymphatic-targeted drug carriers: Study on cell-specific toxicity in vitro and lymphatic targeting in vivo. *J. Mater. Chem. B* **2015**, *3*, 5249–5260. [CrossRef]
67. Vimala, K.; Shanthi, K. Synergistic effect of chemo-photothermal for breast cancer therapy using folic acid (FA) modified zinc oxide nanosheet. *J. Colloid Interface Sci.* **2017**, *488*, 92–108. [CrossRef]
68. Padmanabhan, J.; Kyriakides, T.R. Nanomaterials, Inflammation, and Tissue Engineering. *Wires Nanomater. Nanobiotechnol.* **2015**, *7*, 355–370. [CrossRef]
69. Bhowmick, S.; Rother, S. Biomimetic electrospun scaffolds from main extracellular matrix components for skin tissue engineering application – The role of chondroitin sulfate and sulfated hyaluronan. *Mater. Sci. Eng. C* **2017**, *79*, 15–22. [CrossRef]
70. Jiang, Y.C.; Jiang, L. Electrospun polycaprolactone/gelatin composites with enhanced cell–matrix interactions as blood vessel endothelial layer scaffolds. *Mater. Sci. Eng. C* **2017**, *71*, 901–908. [CrossRef]
71. Bose, S.; Roy, M. Recent advances in bone tissue engineering scaffolds. *Trends Biotechnol.* **2012**, *30*, 546–554. [CrossRef] [PubMed]
72. Trombetta, R.; Inzana, J.A. 3D Printing of Calcium Phosphate Ceramics for Bone Tissue Engineering and Drug Delivery. *Ann. Biomed. Eng.* **2017**, *45*, 23–44. [CrossRef] [PubMed]
73. Felice, B.; Sanchez, M.A. Controlled degradability of PCL-ZnO nanofibrous scaffolds for bone tissue engineering and their antibacterial activity. *Mater. Sci. Eng. C* **2018**, *93*, 724–738. [CrossRef] [PubMed]
74. Park, J.K.; Kim, Y.J. The Topographic Effect of Zinc Oxide Nanoflowers on Osteoblast Growth and Osseointegration. *Adv. Mater.* **2010**, *22*, 4857–4861. [CrossRef] [PubMed]
75. Padovani, G.C.; Feitosa, V.P. Advances in Dental Materials through Nanotechnology: Facts, Perspectives and Toxicological Aspects. *Trends Biotechnol.* **2015**, *33*, 621–636. [CrossRef] [PubMed]
76. Ciofani, G.; Genchi, G.G. ZnO nanowire arrays as substrates for cell proliferation and differentiation. *Mater. Sci. Eng. C* **2012**, *32*, 341–347. [CrossRef]
77. Errico, V.; Arrabito, G. High-Density ZnO Nanowires as a Reversible Myogenic–Differentiation Switch. *Acs Appl. Mater. Interfaces* **2018**, *10*, 14097–14107. [CrossRef] [PubMed]
78. Follmann, D.M.; Naves, A.F. Hybrid Materials and Nanocomposites as Multifunctional Biomaterials. *Curr. Pharm. Des.* **2017**, *23*, 3794–3813. [CrossRef]
79. Jun, I.; Han, H.S. Electrospun Fibrous Scaffolds for Tissue Engineering: Viewpoints on Architecture and Fabrication. *Int. J. Mol. Sci.* **2018**, *19*, 745. [CrossRef]
80. Fang, J.; Wang, X. Functional applications of electrospun nanofibers. In *Nanofibers—Production, Properties and Functional Applications*; InTech—Open Access Publisher: London, UK, 2011; pp. 287–326.
81. Therona, S.A.; Zussmanab, E. Experimental investigation of the governing parameters in the electrospinning of polymer solutions. *Polymer* **2004**, *45*, 2017–2030. [CrossRef]
82. Soliman, S.; Pagliari, S. Multiscale three-dimensional scaffolds for soft tissue engineering via multimodal electrospinning. *Acta Biomater.* **2006**, *6*, 1227–1237. [CrossRef] [PubMed]
83. Wannatong, L.; Sirivat, A. Effects of solvents on electrospun polymeric fibers: Preliminary study on polystyrene. *Polym. Int.* **2004**, *53*, 1851–1859. [CrossRef]
84. Luo, C.J.; Nangrejo, M. A novel method of selecting solvents for polymer electrospinning. *Polymer* **2010**, *51*, 1654–1662. [CrossRef]
85. Liverani, L.; Boccaccini, A.R. Versatile Production of Poly(Epsilon-Caprolactone) Fibers by Electrospinning Using Benign Solvents. *Nanomaterials* **2016**, *6*, 75. [CrossRef] [PubMed]

86. Dotivala, A.C.; Puthuveetil, K.P. Shear Force Fiber Spinning: Process Parameter and Polymer Solution Property Consideration. *Polymers* **2019**, *11*, 294. [CrossRef]
87. Shin, D.; Kim, J. Experimental study on jet impact speed in near-field electrospinning for precise patterning of nanofiber. *J. Manuf. Process.* **2018**, *36*, 231–237. [CrossRef]
88. Hekmati, A.H.; Rashidi, A. Effect of needle length, electrospinning distance, and solution concentration on morphological properties of polyamide-6 electrospun nanowebs. *Text. Res. J.* **2013**, *83*. [CrossRef]
89. Asghari, F.; Samiei, M. Biodegradable and biocompatible polymers for tissue engineering application: A review. *Artif. Cells Nanomed. Biotechnol.* **2017**, *45*, 185–192. [CrossRef]
90. Malikmammadov, E.; Tanir, T.E. PCL and PCL-based materials in biomedical applications. *J. Biomater. Sci. Polym. Ed.* **2018**, *29*, 863–893. [CrossRef] [PubMed]
91. Munchow, E.A.; Albuquerque, M.T.P. Development and characterization of novel ZnO-loaded electrospun membranes for periodontal regeneration. *Dent. Mater.* **2015**, *31*, 1038–1051. [CrossRef] [PubMed]
92. Sezer, U.A.; Ozturk, K. Zero valent zinc nanoparticles promote neuroglial cell proliferation: A biodegradable and conductive filler candidate for nerve regeneration. *J. Mater. Sci. Mater. Med.* **2017**, *28*.
93. Augustine, R.; Dominic, E.A. Investigation of angiogenesis and its mechanism using zinc oxide nanoparticle-loaded electrospun tissue engineering scaffolds. *Rsc Adv.* **2014**, *4*, 51528–51536. [CrossRef]
94. Li, Y.; Sun, L. The Investigation of ZnO/Poly(vinylidene fluoride) Nanocomposites with Improved Mechanical, Piezoelectric, and Antimicrobial Properties for Orthopedic Applications. *J. Biomed. Nanotechnol.* **2018**, *14*, 536–545. [CrossRef] [PubMed]
95. Lee, Y.S.; Collins, G. Neurite extension of primary neurons on electrospun piezoelectric scaffolds. *Acta Biomater.* **2011**, *7*, 3877–3886. [CrossRef] [PubMed]
96. Augustine, R.; Dan, P. Electrospun poly(vinylidene fluoride-trifluoroethylene)/zinc oxide nanocomposite tissue engineering scaffolds with enhanced cell adhesion and blood vessel formation. *Nano Res.* **2017**, *10*, 3358–3376. [CrossRef]
97. Amna, T.; Hassan, M.S. Zinc oxide-doped poly(urethane) spider web nanofibrous scaffold via one-step electrospinning: A novel matrix for tissue engineering. *Appl. Microbiol. Biotechnol.* **2013**, *97*, 1725–1734. [CrossRef] [PubMed]
98. Amna, T.; Hassan, M.S. Electrospun nanofibers of ZnO-TiO2 hybrid: Characterization and potential as an extracellular scaffold for supporting myoblasts. *Surf. Interface Anal.* **2014**, *46*, 72–76. [CrossRef]
99. Zhu, P.; Weng, Z. Biomedical Applications of Functionalized ZnO Nanomaterials: From Biosensors to Bioimaging. *Adv. Mater. Interfaces* **2016**, *3*. [CrossRef]
100. Parham, S.; Wicaksono, D.H.B. Antimicrobial Treatment of Different Metal Oxide Nanoparticles: A Critical Review. *J. Chin. Med. Soc.* **2016**, *63*, 385–393. [CrossRef]
101. Häffner, S.M.; Malmsten, M. Membrane interactions and antimicrobial effects of inorganic nanoparticles. *Adv. Colloid Interface Sci.* **2017**, *248*, 105–128. [CrossRef] [PubMed]
102. Eutimio, M.; Monroy, E. Enhanced healing and anti-inflammatory effects of a carbohydrate polymer with zinc oxide in patients with chronic venous leg ulcers: Preliminary results. *Arch. Med. Sci.* **2018**, *14*, 336–344. [CrossRef]
103. Kantipudi, S.; Sunkara, J.R. Enhanced wound healing activity of Ag–ZnO composite NPs in Wistar Albino rats. *Iet Digit. Libr.* **2018**, *12*, 473–478. [CrossRef] [PubMed]
104. Lu, Z.; Gao, J. Enhanced antibacterial and wound healing activities of microporous chitosan-Ag/ZnO composite dressing. *Carbohydr. Polym.* **2017**, *156*, 460–469. [CrossRef] [PubMed]
105. Khorasani, M.T.; Joorabloo, A. Incorporation of ZnO nanoparticles into heparinised polyvinyl alcohol/chitosan hydrogels for wound dressing application. *Int. J. Biol. Macromol.* **2018**, *114*, 1203–1215. [CrossRef] [PubMed]
106. Zhai, M.; Xu, Y. Keratin-chitosan/n-ZnO nanocomposite hydrogel for antimicrobial treatment of burn wound healing: Characterization and biomedical application. *J. Photochem. Photobiol. B Biol.* **2018**, *180*, 253–258. [CrossRef] [PubMed]
107. Chhabra, H.; Deshpande, R. A nano zinc oxide doped electrospun scaffold improves wound healing in a rodent model. *Rsc Adv.* **2016**, *6*, 1428–1439. [CrossRef]
108. Shalumon, K.T.; Anulekha, K.H. Sodium alginate/poly(vinyl alcohol)/nano ZnO composite nanofibers for antibacterial wound dressings. *Int. J. Biol. Macromol.* **2011**, *49*, 247–254. [CrossRef]

109. Augustine, R.; Dominic, E.A. Electrospun polycaprolactone membranes incorporated with ZnO nanoparticles as skin substitutes with enhanced fibroblast proliferation and wound healing. *Rsc Adv.* **2014**, *4*, 24777–24785. [CrossRef]
110. Abdalkarim, S.Y.H.; Yu, H.Y. Electrospun poly(3-hydroxybutyrate-co-3-hydroxy-valerate)/cellulose reinforced nanofibrous membranes with ZnO nanocrystals for antibacterial wound dressings. *Cellulose* **2017**, *24*, 2925–2938. [CrossRef]
111. Ahmed, R.; Tariq, M. Novel electrospun chitosan/polyvinyl alcohol/zinc oxide nanofibrous mats with antibacterial and antioxidant properties for diabetic wound healing. *Int. J. Biol. Macromol.* **2018**, *120*, 385–393. [CrossRef] [PubMed]
112. Rath, G.; Hussain, T. Development and characterization of cefazolin loaded zinc oxide nanoparticles composite gelatin nanofiber mats for postoperative surgical wounds. *Mater. Sci. Eng. C* **2016**, *58*, 242–253. [CrossRef] [PubMed]
113. Li, N.; Zhang, J. Anti-fouling potential evaluation of PVDF membranes modified with ZnO against polysaccharide. *Chem. Eng. J.* **2016**, *304*, 65–174. [CrossRef]
114. Pascariu, P.; Olaru, L. Photocatalytic activity of ZnO nanostructures grown on electrospun CAB ultrafine fibers. *Appl. Surf. Sci.* **2018**, *455*, 61–69. [CrossRef]
115. Pant, B.; Ojha, G.P.O. Fly-ash-incorporated electrospun zinc oxide nanofibers: Potential material for environmental remediation. *Environ. Pollut.* **2019**, *245*, 163–172. [CrossRef] [PubMed]
116. Kunjuzwa, N.; Nthunya, L.N. Chapter 5-The use of nanomaterials in the synthesis of nanofiber membranes and their application in water treatment. In *Advanced Nanomaterials for Membrane Synthesis and its Applications*; Elsevier: Amsterdam, The Netherlands, 2019; pp. 101–125.
117. Mai, Z.; Xiong, Z. Multifunctionalization of cotton fabrics with polyvinylsilsesquioxane/ZnO composite coatings. *Carbohydr. Polym.* **2018**, *199*, 516–525. [CrossRef]
118. Song, K.; Wu, Q. 20-Electrospun nanofibers with antimicrobial properties. In *Electrospun Nanofibers*; Woodhead Publishing Series in Textiles; Woodhead Publishing: Cambridge, UK, 2017; pp. 551–569.
119. Mallakpour, S.; Behranvand, V. Nanocomposites based on biosafe nano ZnO and different polymeric matrixes for antibacterial, optical, thermal and mechanical applications. *Eur. Polym. J.* **2016**, *84*, 377–403. [CrossRef]
120. Li, X.; Xing, Y. Antimicrobial activities of ZnO powder coated PVC film to inactivate food pathogens. *Int. J. Food Sci. Technol.* **2009**, *44*, 2161–2168. [CrossRef]
121. Ejaz, M.; Arfat, Y.A. Zinc oxide nanorods/clove essential oil incorporated Type B gelatin composite films and its applicability for shrimp packaging. *Food Packag. Shelf Life* **2018**, *15*, 113–121. [CrossRef]
122. Espitia, P.J.P.; Soares, N.F.F. Zinc Oxide Nanoparticles: Synthesis, Antimicrobial Activity and Food Packaging Applications. *Food Bioprocess. Technol.* **2012**, *5*, 1447–1464. [CrossRef]
123. Wang, Z.; Zhang, L. The Antibacterial Polyamide 6-ZnO Hierarchical Nanofibers Fabricated by Atomic Layer Deposition and Hydrothermal Growth. *Nanoscale Res. Lett.* **2017**, *12*. [CrossRef] [PubMed]
124. Prone, G.P.; Bermudez, P.S. Enhanced antibacterial nanocomposite mats by coaxial electrospinning of polycaprolactone fibers loaded with Zn-based nanoparticles. *Nanomed. Nanotechnol. Biol. Med.* **2018**, *14*, 1695–1706. [CrossRef] [PubMed]
125. Anitha, S.; Brabu, B. Optical, bactericidal and water repellent properties of electrospun nano-composite membranes of cellulose acetate and ZnO. *Carbohydr. Polym.* **2013**, *97*, 856–863. [CrossRef] [PubMed]
126. Kima, H.; Joshi, M.K. Polydopamine-assisted immobilization of hierarchical zinc oxide nanostructures on electrospun nanofibrous membrane for photocatalysis and antimicrobial activity. *J. Colloid Interface Sci.* **2018**, *513*, 566–574. [CrossRef] [PubMed]
127. Malwal, D.; Gopinath, P. Efficient adsorption and antibacterial properties of electrospun CuO-ZnO composite nanofibers for water remediation. *J. Hazard. Mater.* **2017**, *321*, 611–621. [CrossRef] [PubMed]
128. Liu, Y.; Li, Y. Hydrophobic Ethylcellulose/Gelatin Nanofibers Containing Zinc Oxide Nanoparticles for Antimicrobial Packaging. *J. Agric. Food Chem.* **2018**, *66*, 9498–9506. [CrossRef] [PubMed]

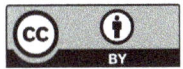

© 2019 by the authors. Licensee MDPI, Basel, Switzerland. This article is an open access article distributed under the terms and conditions of the Creative Commons Attribution (CC BY) license (http://creativecommons.org/licenses/by/4.0/).

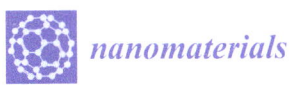

Article

Inhibition of Wild *Enterobacter cloacae* Biofilm Formation by Nanostructured Graphene- and Hexagonal Boron Nitride-Coated Surfaces

Elsie Zurob [1,2], Geraldine Dennett [1], Dana Gentil [1], Francisco Montero-Silva [1], Ulrike Gerber [3], Pamela Naulín [4], Andrea Gómez [4], Raúl Fuentes [5], Sheila Lascano [6], Thiago Henrique Rodrigues da Cunha [7], Cristian Ramírez [8], Ricardo Henríquez [9], Valeria del Campo [9], Nelson Barrera [4], Marcela Wilkens [2] and Carolina Parra [1,*]

1. Laboratorio Nanobiomateriales, Departamento de Física, Universidad Técnica Federico Santa María, Avenida España 1680, Valparaíso, Chile; elsie.zurob@usach.cl (E.Z.); g.dennett@gmail.com (G.D.); dana.gentil@usm.cl (D.G.); monteroster@gmail.com (F.M.-S.)
2. Laboratorio de Microbiología Básica y Aplicada, Universidad de Santiago de Chile, Avenida Libertador Bernardo O'Higgins 3363, Santiago, Chile; marcela.wilkens@usach.cl
3. Faculty Environment and Natural Science, Institute of Biotechnology, Brandenburg University of Technology, Universitätsplatz 1, 01968 Senftenberg, Germany; gerberu@b-tu.de
4. Facultad de Ciencias Biológicas, Pontificia Universidad Católica de Chile, Alameda 340, Santiago, Chile; pnaulin@uc.cl (P.N.); agomez@bio.puc.cl (A.G.); nbarrera@bio.puc.cl (N.B.)
5. Departamento de Industrias, Universidad Técnica Federico Santa María, Avenida España 1680, Valparaíso, Chile; raul.fuentes@usm.cl
6. Departamento de Mecánica, Universidad Técnica Federico Santa María, Avda. Vicuña Mackenna 3939, Santiago, Chile; sheila.lascano@usm.cl
7. Departamento de Física, CTNanotubos, Universidade Federal de Minas Gerais, Belo Horizonte 31310260, Brazil; thiago.cunha@ctnano.com.br
8. Departamento de Ingeniería Química y Ambiental, Universidad Técnica Federico Santa María, Avenida España 1680, Valparaíso, Chile; cristian.ramirez@usm.cl
9. Departamento de Física, Universidad Técnica Federico Santa María, Avenida España 1680, Valparaíso, Chile; ricardo.henriquez@usm.cl (R.H.); valeria.delcampo@usm.cl (V.d.C.)
* Correspondence: carolina.parra@usm.cl

Received: 7 December 2018; Accepted: 25 December 2018; Published: 2 January 2019

Abstract: Although biofilm formation is a very effective mechanism to sustain bacterial life, it is detrimental in medical and industrial sectors. Current strategies to control biofilm proliferation are typically based on biocides, which exhibit a negative environmental impact. In the search for environmentally friendly solutions, nanotechnology opens the possibility to control the interaction between biological systems and colonized surfaces by introducing nanostructured coatings that have the potential to affect bacterial adhesion by modifying surface properties at the same scale. In this work, we present a study on the performance of graphene and hexagonal boron nitride coatings (h-BN) to reduce biofilm formation. In contraposition to planktonic state, we focused on evaluating the efficiency of graphene and h-BN at the irreversible stage of biofilm formation, where most of the biocide solutions have a poor performance. A wild *Enterobacter cloacae* strain was isolated, from fouling found in a natural environment, and used in these experiments. According to our results, graphene and h-BN coatings modify surface energy and electrostatic interactions with biological systems. This nanoscale modification determines a significant reduction in biofilm formation at its irreversible stage. No bactericidal effects were found, suggesting both coatings offer a biocompatible solution for biofilm and fouling control in a wide range of applications.

Keywords: graphene; h-BN; nanostructured coatings; biofilms; *E. cloacae*

1. Introduction

Under natural conditions, microorganisms often encounter complex and hostile environments [1]. Their ability to quickly adapt to these changes in their surroundings will ensure their survival. The activation of survival mechanisms in bacteria relies on their ability to form communities called biofilms [2]. These mechanisms allow bacteria to attach to surfaces through the secretion of exopolymeric substances (EPS) [3], generating a three-dimensional enclosed matrix [4] composed mainly of polysaccharides, proteins, and DNA [5,6]. Biofilm formation provides bacteria with a defense against predators and chemical toxins; such as biocides and antibiotics [7].

Bacteria within biofilms are more resistant than those in planktonic or sessile state. Studies have shown that biofilm cells can tolerate up to 1000 times more antibiotic concentrations than their planktonic counterparts, and are even able to survive in environments exposed to biocides and UV radiation [8]. This makes it very hard to eradicate them once they have reached their biofilm form [9].

Although biofilm formation is a very effective mechanism for sustaining bacterial life, at the same time, it is unfavorable and harmful in human environments; such as in the medical field (where biofilms are responsible for at least 65% of all bacterial infections [8]), in food processing areas (where they lead to food spoilage [10]), and industrial sectors (where they increase fuel and energy consumption, and cause important economic losses [2,11,12]). In addition, biofilms have been linked to the proliferation of highly invasive freshwater microalgae such as *Didymosphenia geminate* (rock snot) [13].

Currently, these issues are addressed using biocides, which are chemical agents with antiseptic, disinfectant, or preservative properties used to control and prevent biofilm formation. The use of biocides does not only have an economic impact, but also is responsible for harmful by-products, many being toxic and even carcinogenic [14]. Biocides such as tributyltin (TBT), copper pyrithione (CuPT), triclosan [15], and quaternary ammonium compounds [16], have a severe impact on marine environments due to their high toxicity [11]. Chlorine is one of the most common antimicrobial agents used to control microorganisms, however, studies have shown that its efficiency applies mostly to planktonic bacteria causing a mild effect on biofilms [17].

In fact, it is important to highlight that a vast majority of studies regarding biofilm control and prevention have been performed on planktonic cells rather than biofilm cells (European Standard—EN 1276:2009). This misconception leads to the current ineffective results obtained by conventional cleaning and disinfection strategies [2].

Understanding biofilm formation might open the possibility to investigate new alternatives to control, or reduce its impact on surfaces. Biofilm formation begins when planktonic cells interact with surfaces establishing a *reversible* first adhesion [18]. At this stage, the ability of bacteria to attach to a surface is dictated by the presence of appendages and associated proteins in the surface of the cells. Once the initial electrostatic repulsion between cell and surface is overcome, the *irreversible* attachment begins [19]. This attachment is mediated by the secretion of polysaccharides and the production of adhesins [18].

All these interactions between surface and cell occur at a nanometric level. Interesting approaches have been introduced to control biofilm formation and bacterial development on surfaces by intervening at this particular nanometric scale [20]. One example of this is surface modifications with specific and highly controlled nanotextures; such as regular nanopatterns [21], which affect biofilm formation and development. However, surface patterning techniques are in their early development and very expensive.

Another nanoscale strategy consists of the use of nanomaterials and nanostructured coatings. A widely studied nanomaterial is graphene oxide (GO), which possesses a strong antimicrobial effect [22,23], due to the cell membrane disruption caused by its interaction with the functional groups present in this nanomaterial. This cytotoxic effect on bacterial cells also presents a potential risk to human health and the environment [24]. A similar effect on biofilms has also been described for silver nanomaterials and multi-walled carbon nanotubes [25–27]. Finally, nanoparticles of copper oxide

(CuO) are usually used to reinforce antifouling paintings, in spite of its high toxicity [28] and harmful impact on marine environments and aquatic species [11].

To date, there is no known technique that successfully prevents or controls biofilms without causing adverse side effects [2]. Within this context, the search for new strategies must continue. One of the most recently developed nanomaterials is single-layer graphene, which has been poorly investigated for biofilm-control applications. Single-layer graphene (SLG) is usually produced by chemical vapor deposition, and is composed of a single-atom-thick sheet of sp^2-bonded carbon atoms arranged in a honeycomb two-dimensional lattice [29]. Chemical vapor deposition (CVD) graphene is the most popular form of large-area graphene and reaches surface areas in the centimeters square range.

In contrast, Graphene Oxide (GO) coatings are primarily obtained by chemical oxidation of graphite [30], and it can be defined as a graphene flake with carboxylic groups at its edges, and phenol hydroxyl and epoxide groups on its basal plane [31]. This range of reactive oxygen functional groups confers antimicrobial activity and toxicity mechanisms, linked to oxidative stress [29,32]. Unlike GO coatings, SLG coatings do not possess bactericide activity, although a previous study using planktonic bacteria has shown that SLG interferes with the genetic expression of bacterial adhesion [33]. This study shows that SLG coatings considerably reduce the adhesion of bacteria in planktonic state (floating cells) and sessile state (attached cells without EPS production) due to surface interaction modification [34]. Such an initial biofilm growth stage was tuned by evaluating bacterial adhesion to SLG-coated surfaces at a short time (24 h). However, SGL coating efficiency to control the formation of biofilms at its advanced *irreversible* stage (which is, in fact, the most complex form to eradicate) has not been explored yet.

Recently, a new generation of graphene-like two-dimensional materials with an atomic structure similar to graphene, but different chemical composition and properties, have attracted widespread attention [35]. One of them, hexagonal boron nitride (h-BN), has shown similar biological performance to SLG under microbial corrosion conditions [36]. h-BN is composed of boron and nitrogen atoms in a honeycomb arrangement, consisting of sp^2-bonded two dimensional layers [37]. There is a similarity in structure with graphene; as atoms are bound by strong covalent bonds, forming a single h-BN layer. But unlike the highly conductive graphene, h-BN possesses a wide band gap of 6 eV [38]. Such differences (and similarities) between h-BN and SGL properties could help to elucidate any connection between the interaction of graphitic-like membranes and biological systems. In particular, the lack of information regarding nanotechnological approaches to control biofilm formation at its *irreversible* stage motivated us to study the efficiency of SLG and h-BN coatings to prevent biofilm formation at such growth conditions, in contrast to planktonic or sessile state bacteria (*reversible* growth stage).

As a bacterial model, a wild strain of *Enterobacter cloacae* isolated from natural environments was selected. *Enterobacter cloacae* is a Gram-negative bacterium that belongs to the family *Enterobacteriaceae*. It has been reported that it forms biofilms in most environments, causing opportunistic infections and colonizing medical devices, being one of the ten most isolated nosocomial pathogens [10,39]. Their ability to persist in these environments, as well as their virulence, makes them a suitable model for this study. To evaluate the efficiency of SLG and h-BN coatings, we first determined the growth time at which *E. cloacae* reaches its *irreversible* biofilm stage. At that particular time the effect of those coatings on biofilm formation was studied.

2. Materials and Methods

2.1. Synthesis and Transfer

Single-layer graphene growth (for transferred samples) was performed through chemical vapor deposition (CVD) with methane as a precursor, using 25 μm thick copper foil (99.99% purity) as a synthesis substrate. The CVD growth process was performed inside a quartz tubular furnace after heating at 1000 °C under a methane-hydrogen flow rate of 20 sccm (standard cubic centimeter per minute) and 10 sccm, respectively, as reported by Parra et al. [33]. A slight modification of this methodology was introduced by supplying this mixed flux in five steps of 20 min each. Between each step, the sample was held only under the hydrogen flux for 10 min to ensure a high coverage. The final methane step was followed by rapid cooling under a hydrogen-argon flux of 10 sccm and 20 sccm, respectively. Commercial single-layer h-BN grown on Cu foil were used for this study (Graphene Supermarket, Calverton, NY, USA). The PMMA (Polymethyl methacrylate)-assisted transfer method was used in order to obtain transferred graphene and h-BN on glass [36] (See supplementary Figure S1). All graphene and h-BN samples used in this study were 1 cm^2 in area.

2.2. Characterization SLG and h-BN

Scanning tunnelling microscopy (STM; UHV-VT Omicron, Uppsala, Sweden) and atomic force microscopy (AFM; Asylum Research Instruments MFP-3D, Santa Barbara, CA, USA) were used to characterize the topography of samples with nanoscale resolution. MicroRaman measurements (Renishaw, 532 nm laser, Gloucestershire, UK) were used to characterize the quality of as-grown and transferred graphene and h-BN. Contact angle measurements were performed to characterize surface hydrophobicity of coated and uncoated samples. A drop of Milli-Q water (2 µL) was placed on the surface of graphene- and h-BN-coated glass samples, and images were immediately captured using a high-resolution camera. The contact angle was measured based on image analysis [40] using the image processing software Image J with the plug-in Drop Shape Analysis (bundled with 64-bit Java 1.6.0_24, public domain) based on B-spline snakes algorithm [41].

2.3. Strain Isolation

Enterobacter cloacae strain used in this study was isolated from biofilm samples collected from aquaculture nettings off of the coast of Castro, Región de Los Lagos, Chile. This bacterial strain was isolated using the streak plate method. The sample was grown overnight on marine broth (MB) (BD Difco Marine broth 2216, NJ, USA) at 28 °C for 18 h, and spectrophotometrically standardized to reach a final absorbance of 0.1 at 600 nm (Thermo Scientific Multiskan GO, Waltham, MA, USA).

This *E. cloacae* strain was selected based upon its ability to form biofilm following the the microtiter assay described by O'Toole [42]. To identify the *E. cloacae* strain, multiple assays were conducted. Cellular morphology and biochemical tests were evaluated [43,44] (See supplementary data, Table S1). In addition, molecular identification based on the 16S rDNA sequence was accomplished using a DNA extraction and purification kit (FavorPrep™ Soil DNA Isolation Mini Kit, Wembley, Australia). Gene 16S rRNA was amplified using primers F799 [45] and R1492 [46] synthesized by Integrated DNA Technologies, USA (Fermelo Biotec, Santiago, Chile). The amplified products were sequenced (Macrogen, Seoul, Korea), and analyzed using Mega6 and Basic Local Alignment Search Tool (BLAST) software (2.6.0, Rockville, MD, USA) (https://blast.ncbi.nlm.nih.gov/Blast.cgi).

2.4. Biofilm Formation Microtiter Assay—Biofilm Growth over Time

E. cloacae biofilm formation was measured using a modification of the standard method described by O'Toole [42]. Five milliliters of MB were inoculated with an isolated colony and grown overnight at 28 °C. Before use, the bacterial suspension was diluted to reach a final optical density (OD 600) of 0.1. A volume of 20 µL of the standardized inoculum was pipetted into a sterile, polystyrene 96-well flat-bottomed microtiter plate (Cell culture plate, Nest Biotech Co., Ltd., Wuxi, China) containing 180 µL of MB. A 200 µL aliquot of the diluted bacterial suspension was added to each growth control well. The negative control wells contained 200 µL of broth medium only. The plate was incubated aerobically at 28 °C for different periods of time (24, 48, 72, and 96 h). The culture medium was refreshed in one set of samples every 24 h. After incubation, the culture media was carefully removed from the wells and washed three times with 200 µL of phosphate-buffered saline (PBS) to remove the non-adherent bacteria.

The plates were then left to air dry under sterile laminar flow in a safety biosecurity cabinet (Nuaire NU-425 Class II, Type A2, Plymouth, MN, USA) for 1 h. Cells adhered to the plate were stained with 200 µL of 0.1% (w/v) crystal violet (Merck, Damm, Germany) for 30 min. The plates were carefully rinsed off under running tap water to remove excess stain, and air-dried under sterile laminar flow at room temperature. Bound dye was dissolved with 200 µL of 95% (v/v) ethanol. The optical density (OD) of each well was measured at 590 nm using a microtiter plate reader (Thermo Scientific Multiskan™ GO Microplate Spectrophotometer), using ethanol 95% as blank. To quantify the biofilm formed on each experiment, six replica wells were used per experiment and three independent experiments were performed.

2.5. Colored Staining in Bright Light Microscopy—Effect of Media Replacement on Biofilm Growth

A 100 µL inoculum of E. cloacae strain suspension (OD_{600nm} at 0.1) was transferred to a glass coverslip (18 mm × 18 mm, Sail Brand, Haimen, China) and incubated in a sterile petri dish at 25 °C for different periods of time (24, 48, 72, and 96 h). Two different sets of samples were carried out separately; one with media replacement every 24 h, and the other set with no media replacement. After the corresponding incubation time, safranin staining, Alcian blue/safranin staining, and Gram staining were performed on the samples, separately. The samples were observed by bright-field microscopy on the 100× objective lens (Carl Zeiss Axiostar Plus Transmitted-Light Microscope, Oerzen, Germany).

2.6. Inhibition of Biofilm Growth in Coated Surfaces

A 100 µL inoculum of standardized E. cloacae bacterial suspension was transferred to a 1 × 1 cm² coated glass samples (microscope slides Cat No. 7105, Sail Brand, China); graphene-coated glass, h-BN-coated glass, and uncoated glass (triplicate test for all samples). Samples were incubated in a sterile petri dish at 28 °C for 48 h. Marine broth media was replaced on all samples at 24 h. Once the incubation period had elapsed, media was removed, and samples were washed in sequence with sterile water, phosphate buffered saline (PBS), and sterile water. Once the samples were completely dried under sterile laminar flow, 100 µL of 0.1% crystal violet solution was pipetted on the surface and samples were incubated for 30 min at room temperature. Unbound dye was removed by several rinses with sterile water until no more dye was solubilized. Samples were air dried under sterile laminar flow. Once completely dry, samples were transferred to a 6-well cell culture plate (TrueLine cell culture plate TR5000 6 well, polystyrene, sterile, non-pyrogenic, San Jose, CA, USA), and adhered dye was solubilized with 100 µL of ethanol 95% (Merck, Germany). The rinsed solution was pipetted onto a sterile 96-well (Cell culture plate, Nest Biotech Co., Ltd., China). The optical density (OD) of each well was measured at 590 nm using a microtiter plate reader (Thermo Scientific Multiskan™ GO Microplate Spectrophotometer), using 95% ethanol as blank. To quantify the biofilm formed on each experiment, six replica wells were used per experiment and three independent experiments were performed.

2.7. Scanning Electron Microscopy Images

Scanning electron microscopy (SEM) (Carl Zeiss, EVO MA-10) was used to visually evaluate the architecture of biofilms and coated surfaces with microscale resolution. A 100 µL inoculum of standardized E. cloacae bacterial suspension was transferred to graphene-coated glass, h-BN-coated glass, and uncoated glass (triplicate evaluation for all samples). Samples were incubated in a sterile petri dish (90 mm × 15 mm, Cat. No. 752001, Nest Biotech Co., Ltd., China) at 28 °C for 48 h. Growth media was replaced on all samples at 24 h. Once the incubation period had elapsed, media was removed, and samples were washed sequentially with sterile water, PBS, and sterile water. Samples were air-dried under sterile laminar flow. Samples were fixed with 3.0% (w/v) glutaraldehyde solution for 24 h. The samples were dehydrated by washing with a graded ethanol series (from 10% to 100%) for 3 min each, followed by critical-point drying and gold coating. Scanning Electron Microscopy (SEM) images were recorded using a Carl Zeiss microscope (EVO MA-10).

2.8. Epifluorescence Essay

An inoculum of *E. cloacae* bacterial suspension was transferred onto graphene-coated glass, h-BN-coated glass, and uncoated glass samples (triplicate evaluation for all samples), and incubated following the procedure described in Section 2.6. After the incubation media was removed and samples were washed with sterile water and PBS, and dried under sterile laminar flow. Epifluorescence assays were performed using the L7012 Live/Dead backlight bacterial viability kit protocol. Samples were submerged into solutions provided in the same kit (0.01 mM of Syto9 and 0.06 mM of propidium iodide). Samples were kept in the dark for 15 min and then observed under a fluorescent optical microscopy (Carl Zeiss Axiolab A1microscope).

2.9. Viability of Planktonic Cells Assay—State of Non-Attached Bacteria

After 48 h incubation of *E. cloacae* on coated samples, the viability of non-adhered bacteria was quantified. This allows the evaluation of any possible bactericide activity of graphene and h-BN coatings over bacteria in planktonic state (bacteria that did not reach its biofilm *irreversible* growth stage). *E. cloacae* was incubated for 48 h as described in previous sections. After that period, bacteria non-attached to samples (bacteria suspended in media) were recovered using a standard micropipette. Cell viability was determined using the microdot methodology in a trypticase soy agar (TSA) plate [33]. A volume of 20 µL of the bacteria recovered from each sample surface was pipetted into a sterile, polystyrene 96-well flat-bottomed microtiter plate (Cell culture plate, Nest Biotech Co., Ltd., China), containing 180 µL of tryptic soy broth (TSB) and then diluted each sample until obtaining a dilution of 1×10^{-8}. Five µl aliquots of every dilution were inoculated in TSA plates to obtain CFU/mL. Each experimental trial was conducted in triplicate.

3. Results and Discussion

3.1. E. cloacae Biofilm Growth

To evaluate the efficiency of the nanometric coatings on biofilm adhesion, it is necessary to first evaluate the integrity of the biofilm over time. In fact, most studies focus on bacterial adhesion during the first 24 h of contact between the bacteria and surface [47–49], without evaluating if the biofilm has reached its *irreversible* stage (with the presence of EPS) or not. The efficiency of our nanostructured coatings for reduction of biofilm growth required testing under typical conditions for *irreversible* biofilm growth and before biofilm detachment (Figure S2; for details of biofilm growth cycle).

Biofilm growth curve as a function of time can be obtained by means of optical thickness (optical density—OD), measured as intensity reduction of a light beam transmitted through the biofilm, which correlates with biofilm mass. The kinetic growth curves shown in the plot of Figure 1, quantify the adhered biomass on a glass surface over a 96-h period.

Characteristics of the growth media used for bacterial incubation can affect biofilm growth [49]. Considering our experimental conditions; where nutrients in the incubation medium were constantly consumed by bacteria, we explored the effect of biofilm replacement on biofilm growth every 24 h.

The curve in green illustrates the behavior of a biofilm under starvation (no media replacement incubation–WO/R). Simultaneously, the curve in blue depicts the response under media replacement conditions incubation (W/R). Both curves showed similar results during the first 48 h of incubation regardless of the media conditions applied. After this 48-h period of incubation, the curves showed different patterns of behavior. The media replacement condition showed a consistent increment of growth from 48 to 96 h. The no-media replacement condition presented a decrease in growth, which was later reversed at time 96 h.

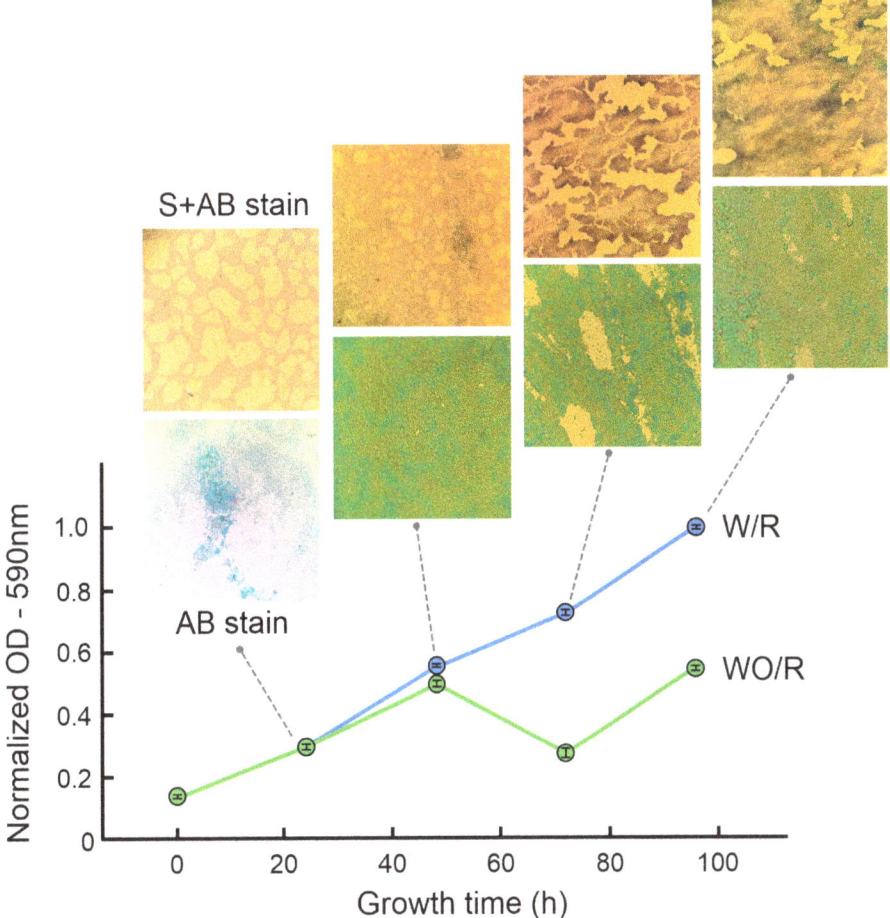

Figure 1. Optical density (OD) measurements and optical micrographs of a staining test of *E. cloacae* biofilms grown on glass as a function of time. The response of biofilm under no-media replacement incubation conditions (WO/R) and media replacement incubation conditions (W/R) is depicted. Corresponding staining test for each time is included (for optical micrographs of staining test for WO/R conditions see supplementary Figure S3).

The difference in the curves' behavior may be explained by the different stages of biofilm development, where stages of detachment may take place after reaching a critical biofilm size. To support this interpretation, we carried out staining tests on the samples at the same growth time as OD analysis. To visualize the architecture of the biofilm, a safranine/Alcian blue staining was used. The presence of exopolysaccharides in the samples was identified using Alcian blue [50]. This staining method is specific for polysaccharide components, and in this case, can be applied to identify the biofilm matrix. Safranine stains bacterial cells in contrast to Alcian blue, which mainly stains EPS [51].

Evaluation of biofilm growth using safranine (S) and Alcian blue (AB) stains (optical microscope images in Figure 1) was in agreement with OD results, showing at 72 h the breakdown of biofilm architecture (EPS and bacteria), presumably connected to biofilm removal by detachment. At 48 h completeness of biofilm was observed using both staining methods, indicating this is the time in the *irreversible* growth stage of biofilm where the maximum biomass size adhered to the surface.

3.2. Morphology of E. cloacae Biofilm at Reversible and Irreversible Stages

To extend the discussion regarding the stage of *E. cloacae* biofilm formation, Figure 2 presents SEM micrographs of glass samples exposed to *E. cloacae* before and at the obtained optimal biofilm growth time.

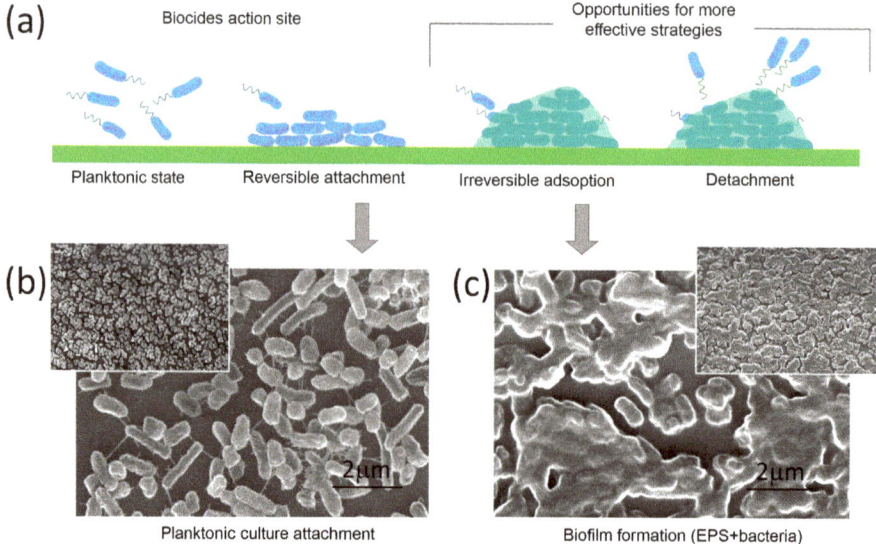

Figure 2. *Enterobacter cloacae* biofilm formation on glass. (**a**) Illustrative diagram of biofilm formation stages: Planktonic state, *reversible* attachment, *irreversible* adsorption, and detachment; (**b**) Scanning electron image (SEM) of *E. cloacae* after 24 h incubation on a glass surface. *Reversible* attachment can be observed by the presence of bacterial surface filaments; and (**c**) SEM image of *E. cloacae* after 48 h incubation on a glass surface. Biofilm formation can be seen by the presence of exopolymeric substances. For more SEM images of biofilm formation stages see Figure S2.

As it was previously discussed, biofilm formation is a complex process, and bacteria must undergo a series of different stages to transform from a planktonic state to *irreversible* adsorption (Figure 2a). Planktonic bacteria following Brownian motion will verge to the surface led by long-range forces [52], the presence of fimbriae and flagella appendages will disrupt the initial electrostatic repulsion between the cell and substratum, and the *reversible* attachment stage will begin. During this phase, bacteria still show Brownian motion and can be easily removed by cleaning [18].

SEM micrograph of the *reversible* attachment stage in the *E. cloacae* biofilm growth (24 h incubation) is shown in Figure 2a. Aggregation and cohesion of bacteria occur, and the presence of bacterial cell appendages (see filaments in SEM image) assists in the attachment of bacteria to the surface or to each other. When these bacterial cells start their transition from this *reversible* to the *irreversible* stage, bacterial cell filaments retract and adhesins mediate attachment by a more intimate contact between bacteria and surface [18]. The *irreversible* attachment finishes when bacteria consolidate the adhesion process by secreting exopolymeric substances. This adhesion to the surface becomes *irreversible*, and bacteria cannot be removed by gentle rinsing [19]. This is clearly observed in Figure 2c (48 h incubation), where the presence of EPS is the critical difference between *reversible* and *irreversible* attachment. In fact, individual bacteria embedded into the EPS wrapping can be distinguished in the SEM micrograph.

This allows identifying the same bacterial concentration (density) over the glass surface in both, the *reversible* (Figure 2b) and *irreversible* stage (Figure 2c).

This qualitative microscopy analysis again confirmed data presented in Figure 1, which indicated that a growth time of 24 h led to an under-incubated biofilm for adhesion experiments. These results indicated that a 48-h incubation time has to be chosen when working with E. cloacae in order to be in its *irreversible* adhesion regime but without presenting detachment for over-incubation. Any assays to demonstrate the effect on biofilm formation of coated surfaces must consider this for the design of the experimental conditions.

3.3. Characterization of Nanostructured Coated Samples

Characterization of as-grown h-BN and SLG on Cu, h-BN, and SLG samples transferred onto glass was performed (Figure 3). The terms graphene or SLG will be used interchangeably. The microstructure was evaluated using scanning electron microscopy (SEM) and atomic force microscopy (AFM) whereas topography (with atomic and nanometric resolution), graphitic quality and composition were evaluated through a combination of scanning tunneling microscopy (STM) and Raman spectroscopy.

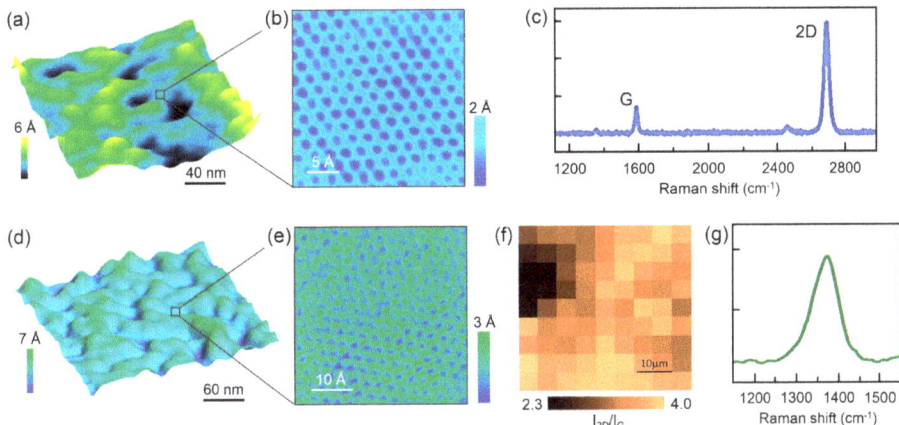

Figure 3. Characterization of h-BN and graphene coatings. (**a**) Atomic force microscopy image of SLG transferred onto glass; (**b**) Scanning tunneling microscopy atomic-resolved image of SLG; (**c**) representative Raman spectrum of SLG; (**d**) STM image of h-BN; (**e**) STM atomic-resolved image of h-BN; (**f**) Raman map of SLG; and (**g**) representative Raman spectrum of h-BN.

Cells of most strains of bacteria are typically 1 micrometer in diameter. Surface roughness on the µm or larger scale and topography irregularities serve as 'hideouts' from unfavorable environments. At the same time, they provide a larger surface area, hence higher hosting capacity, and enhanced bacteria-substrate interaction [53]. In our case, surface roughness obtained from STM images was less than 1 nm (~0.3 nm) for both graphene- and h-BN-coated samples (see Supplementary Figure S4). Surface roughness at the nanometer scale has been shown to increase adhesion [54], but differences in surface roughness on the order of tens of nanometers has been found to be negligible in comparison to other surface properties such as charge [55].

AFM images of single-layer graphene (SLG) grown on Cu, and transferred onto glass showed less than 1 nm corrugation, which is presumably connected to a strain relaxation mechanism generated during the transfer process (Figure 3a). Similar features were found in h-BN transferred onto glass (Figure 3d). Atomic-resolved images of SLG and h-BN on glass obtained using STM (Figure 3b,e) exhibit the distinctive honeycomb structure with an in-plane lattice parameter of 2.5 Å (for SLG) and 2.4 Å (for h-BN), respectively, consistent with literature values [56,57]. Few signs of surface contamination were found by this atomic-resolved technique.

To verify the graphitic quality of graphene coatings micro-Raman spectroscopy measurements were performed. SLG typically display sharp G (1584 cm^{-1}) and 2D (2680–2693 cm^{-1}) bands (Figure 3c). Micro-Raman spectroscopy mapping was carried out on a 50 µm × 50 µm area of graphene transferred onto glass in order to obtain spatial-resolved information regarding ratio of the intensities I_{2D} and I_G of the bands 2D and G (I_{2D}/I_G) (Figure 3f). It is known that the ratio I_{2D}/I_G is dependent on the number of graphene layers. The ratio I_{2D}/I_G >2 is for monolayer graphene, 2 > I_{2D}/I_G > 1 for bilayer graphene, and I_{2D}/I_G <1 for multilayer graphene [58,59]. SLG transferred onto glass samples always exhibits a I_{2D}/I_G ratio larger than 2, confirming the graphitic quality of the samples. Multiple areas of h-BN samples were analyzed and the representative spectrum is shown in Figure 3g. These results are consistent with single layer h-BN, according to values reported in the literature [60].

3.4. Biofilm Formation on h-BN- and Graphene-Coated Samples

Gram staining tests were performed as a first approach to characterize biofilm formation on coated and uncoated glass samples (Figure 4). A well-known method to quantify adhered biomass is the microtiter assay, which uses crystal violet staining. This test allows an indirect quantification of the adhered biomass, as the optical density of bacterial biofilms stained with this dye indicates the concentration of bacteria, and is used as an index of adherence [42].

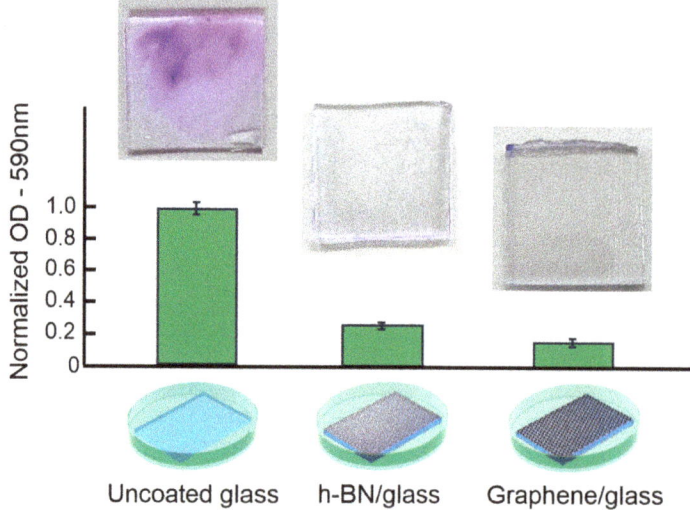

Figure 4. Optical density (OD) and crystal violet results for *E. cloacae* biofilms grown on uncoated glass, h-BN-coated glass, and SLG-coated glass samples.

Figure 4 shows results of optical density for the *E. cloacae* biofilm formed at nanoscale-modified samples after 48 h of exposure. This quantification of biomass formation revealed that graphene-coated glass exhibits 83.6% less biofilm than uncoated glass. In the case of h-BN, a 73.8% suppression of biofilm formation was found. Crystal violet staining results for each sample are also shown in Figure 4. A darker blue color on the uncoated glass surface indicates the effect of the dye staining different layers of the biofilm. Coated glass surfaces showed no apparent coloration under this dye technique, in agreement with the OD results.

Although crystal violet staining quantified the adhered biofilm, it did not give information regarding the state of the cells in the biofilm, as it cannot differentiate between live or dead bacteria.

In order to characterize bacterial adhesion to graphene-coated, h-BN-coated, and uncoated glass samples, SEM and fluorescence microscopy analyses were carried out. Morphology of *E. cloacae* incubated for 48 h on graphene-coated glass, h-BN-coated glass, and uncoated glass samples are shown in Figure 5a,c,e, respectively.

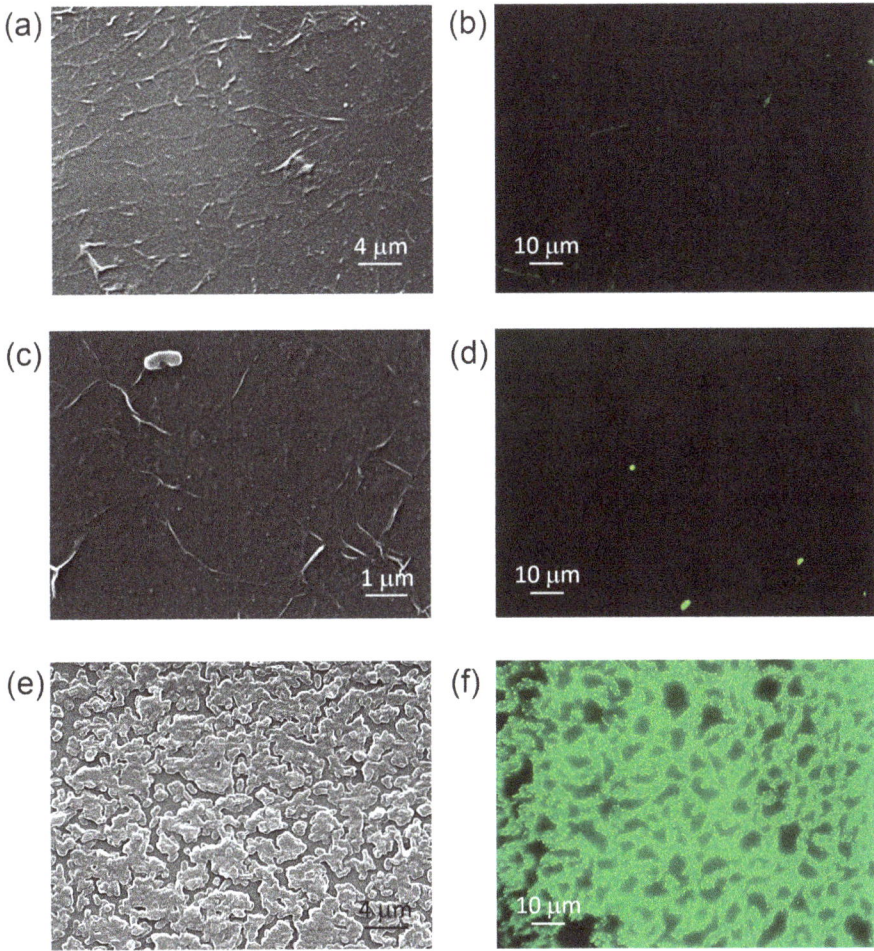

Figure 5. Scanning electron microscopy and epifluorescence images of *Enterobacter cloacae* biofilms' distribution on coated and uncoated glass samples. SEM images of samples after *E. cloacae* 48 h incubation: (**a**) Graphene-coated glass, (**c**) h-BN-coated glass, and (**e**) uncoated glass. Corresponding epifluorescence microscopy micrographs for (**b**) graphene-coated glass, (**d**) h-BN-coated glass, and (**f**) uncoated glass.

SEM images of graphene and h-BN transferred onto glass after 48 h incubation show the absence of attached bacteria or biofilm formation (Figure 5a,c, respectively).

Wrinkles can be identified across the coated samples surface. These structures are usually considered to be a result of compressive stress during cooling caused by the difference in thermal expansion coefficient between two-dimensional layered materials and substrates [38].

After 48 h incubation, the uncoated glass surface was fully covered by *E. cloacae* biofilm, which extended like a percolated network (Figure 5f). Although bacteria were embedded within its extracellular polymeric substances, they still could be individually distinguished (see Figure 2 for comparison).

In order to identify the state of bacteria in such a biofilm structure, epifluorescence microscopy analysis was performed. When using a dead-live kit, green staining is an indication of live bacteria, whereas, red stained bacterial bodies are indicative of dead bacteria. Representative epifluorescence microscopy images of graphene-coated glass, h-BN-coated glass, and uncoated glass samples after 48 h incubation are shown in Figure 5b,d,f, respectively.

Fluorescence microscopy results for uncoated glass samples (Figure 5f) showed that all bacteria present in *E. cloacae* biofilm were in fact alive. In Figure 5b,d, the absence of substantial bacterial adhesion on the graphene-coated and h-BN-coated surfaces concurred with the analyses of OD measured to quantify biofilm formation on these samples. The scarcity in adherence could be related to the inability of these microorganisms to form biofilm (bacteria + EPS) in the presence of these nanostructure-coated surfaces. The lower OD observed in the quantification of biofilm formation and the results obtained by fluorescence microscopy may suggest that bacteria remain in planktonic state, as seen in Figure 2. Fluorescence results for h-BN-coated and graphene-coated glass samples after 48 h of *E. cloacae* incubation were in agreement to SEM images, in terms of the absence of attached bacteria or biofilm. It is important to mention that samples for SEM imaging were prepared through critical-point drying, which applies considerable force on the specimen (present at the phase boundary as the liquid evaporates). This can cause biofilms to detach from the glass surface. Samples for fluorescence imaging, in contrast, do not undergo this aggressive treatment, as it is not needed for this analysis. The absence of bacteria in fluorescence images of coated samples confirms the validity of our SEM results.

Epifluorescence and SEM results suggested both nanostructured coatings suppress dramatically bacterial attachment, which is determinant to biofilm and fouling formation.

To evaluate the state of microorganisms that did not adhere to the nanoscale-modified samples after 48 h, we performed viability tests on the recovered planktonic state bacteria. Recent reports have connected the high-conductance properties of graphene coatings with antibacterial activity [61]. Such effect is claimed to be connected to an increase in the electron exchange between bacteria and graphene. According to our viability results (Figure S5), no bactericide effect was found; neither in recovered planktonic state bacteria (non-adhered bacteria) after exposition to graphene (conducting), nor after exposure to h-BN (insulating). This suggested that electrical conductivity of these nanostructured coatings does not induce bactericide activity. Our results also indicated that coating conductivity is not related to the observed inhibition of biofilm formation.

Unlike other nanomaterials such as graphene oxide, which suppress biofilm formation by membrane rupture leading to cell death [23], our viability results indicated that graphene and h-BN coatings have a different inhibition mechanism of biofilm formation, probably related to long-range and medium-range interactions. In the next section, we explore the influence of electrostatic forces and surface energy on bacterial adhesion on coated surfaces as a possible source of the observed inhibition of biofilm formation.

3.5. Nanostructured Coating Effects on Surface Energy and Electrostatic Interaction

As soon as microorganisms reach a surface, they will be attracted or repelled by it, depending on the sum of the different non-specific interactions [62,63]. The first relevant interaction in this system is the one related to long-range electrostatic forces between graphene-coated glass surfaces and cells that might be affecting the initial (and *reversible*) bacterial adhesion process. Charge contributes to bacterial adhesion to either living or inanimate surfaces. It has been suggested that bacteria, when introduced into aqueous suspensions, are always negatively charged [64]. To determine if electrostatic long-range interactions between graphene-coated glass and bacteria contribute to an initial repulsion between bacteria and the graphene-coated substrate, we performed theoretical calculations to obtain electrostatic force $F(r)$ between bacteria and material surface (glass, graphene-coated glass, and h-BN-coated glass) as a function of their separation distance using the expression [65]:

$$F(r) = \frac{2\pi d_1 d_2 \varepsilon \varepsilon_0 \kappa}{d_1 + d_2} \left(\frac{k_B T}{ze}\right)^2 \frac{\phi_1^2 + \phi_2^2 + (2e^{r\kappa}\phi_1\phi_2)}{(e^{r\kappa} + 1)(e^{r\kappa} - 1)}$$

where F is electrostatic force (in N); r is distance between bacteria and surface (in m); d is the radius of bacteria (or glass piece, or graphene-coated glass, or h-BN-coated glass; in m); ε is the dielectric constant of water [66] (78.43 at 25 °C); ε_0 is the permittivity of free space (8.854 × 10^{-12} C/Jm); k_B is Boltzmann's constant (1.381 × 10^{-23} J/K); T is temperature (25 °C); z is the valence of electrolyte ions (1 for NaCl); and e is the charge of an electron (1.602 × 10^{19} C). The inverse Debye length κ describes the thickness of the electrostatic double layer of counter-ions that surrounds charged parts of the system (bacteria or glass) in solution. For monovalent electrolytes (e.g., NaCl), κ^{-1} is given by $0.304/(c)^{1/2}$ (in 1/nm), where c is the concentration of the electrolyte (in mol/L) and contains information of ionic strength of solution [67]. In our case, we evaluate 2% (w/v), concentration of suspension media (marine broth medium). Surface potential ϕ is described by $ze\psi/k_BT$, where ψ is the surface potential of the bacteria, glass piece, graphene-coated glass piece, and h-BN-coated glass piece (in V). The values of the surface potentials of glass piece, graphene-coated glass piece, h-BN-coated glass piece and *Enterobacter* are −55 mV [68], −77 mV [69], −50 mV [70] and −27 mV [71], respectively.

Figure 6a shows the theoretical force-distance relationship for the bacteria-surface system. According to this result, the electrostatic force in this system is expected to be a repulsive and short range (<5 nm). Although electrostatic repulsion between bacteria and glass always increases when the glass is coated with h-BN or graphene, this effect is stronger for graphene-coated surfaces when a bacterium cell approaches the surface.

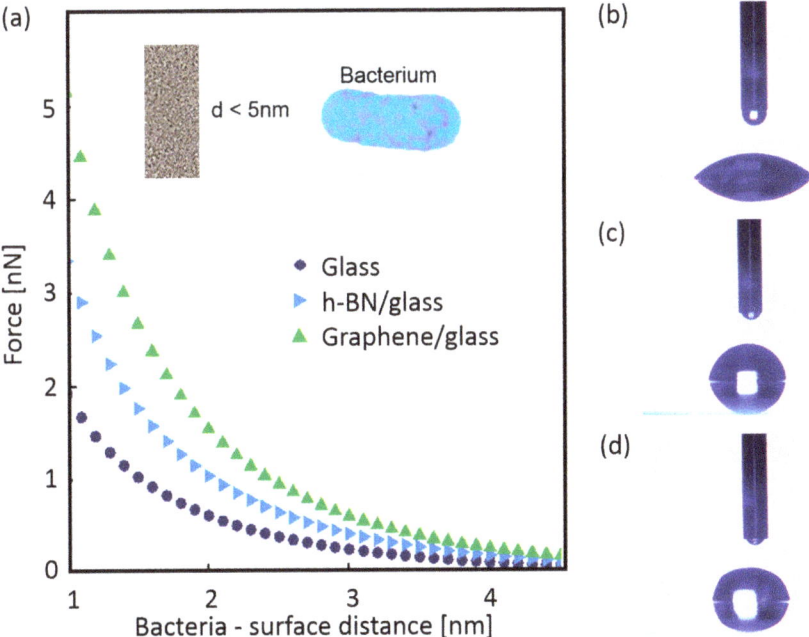

Figure 6. (a) Theoretical calculations of electrostatic force as a function of the distance between bacteria and surface (uncoated and coated glass samples). Images of contact angle measurements for (b) glass, (c) h-BN-coated glass, and (d) graphene-coated glass samples.

An even shorter-range interaction of hydrophobic nature occurs when the bacteria-surface distance is smaller than 1.5 nm (if bacteria are capable of overcoming this initial electrostatic repulsion). Such hydrophobic characteristics are mainly determined by physicochemical surface properties and influence the attachment of bacteria to surfaces [72]. We performed contact angle measurements in order to determine the influence of possible hydrophobic or hydrophilic characteristics of the nanostructured coatings over bacterial adhesion. Figure 6 shows the results for glass (Figure 6b), graphene-coated glass (Figure 6c), and h-BN-coated glass samples (Figure 6d). According to our measurements, a transition from a strongly hydrophilic surface (contact angle of ~42.4° ± 0.7°) for glass substrate to light hydrophilic surface for h-BN-coated glass (contact angle of ~76.8° ± 0.5°), and graphene-coated glass (contact angle of ~81.6° ± 0.3°) was found.

Contact angles are related to the surface free energies [73]. When the contact angle increases (for coated samples), surface wettability decreases (lower surface energy) making it more difficult for the biofilm to spread across the material's surface [74]. These results show that both interactions, electrostatic (<5 nm range) and hydrophobic-hydrophilic (<1.5 nm range), are presumably affecting the bacterial attachment process.

4. Conclusions

We present a study on the performance of graphene and hexagonal boron nitride coatings to reduce *E. cloacae* biofilm formation. In particular, we focused on evaluating their efficiency at the *irreversible* stage of formation (in contraposition to planktonic state), where most of biocide solutions have a poor performance.

According to our experimental and theoretical results, graphene and h-BN coatings modify surface energy and electrostatic interactions with a biological system, which determines a significant reduction in biofilm formation. The fact that the inhibition of biofilms formation is found in both nanostructured coatings (a conducting graphene and an isolating h-BN) indicates electron exchange is not related to this effect.

In addition, no bactericidal effects were found after interaction of the biological system with graphene and h-BN coatings, indicating that the mechanism involved in the inhibition of biofilm formation of such surfaces is not biocidal in nature, like the one used for commercial products designed for this application.

These nanostructured coatings offer an environmentally friendly solution for biofilm and fouling control in a wide range of applications such as the one related to biomedical and industrial sectors. Although international standards regarding biofilm control and prevention are focused on attacking planktonic cells rather than biofilm cells, which is highly ineffective, in this work we provide a successful strategy to reduce biofilm formation which is alternative to biocides and other chemical solutions.

Future work should be focused on evaluating the efficiency of using natural biofilms that are more complex due to their heterogeneous nature.

Supplementary Materials: The following are available online at http://www.mdpi.com/2079-4991/9/1/49/s1, Figure S1: Polymethyl methacrylate (PMMA)-assisted transfer method; Figure S2: Scanning Electron Microscopy images of biofilm growth stages; Figure S3: Optical density (OD) results for biofilms grown with and without media replacement; Figure S4: Roughness analysis of coated glass samples; Figure S5: Cell viability of *E. cloacae* in planktonic state; Table S1: Biochemical test for bacterial strain identification.

Author Contributions: E.Z., M.W., and C.P. designed the experiment; E.Z., D.G., F.M.-S., U.G., P.N., A.G., R.H., S.L., T.H.R.d.C., C.R., V.d.C., M.W., and C.P. carried out the synthesis and characterization of nanomaterials; E.Z. and G.D. carried out the microbiological experiment; E.Z., G.D., M.W., and C.P. analyzed the data and wrote the manuscript; E.Z., G.D., M.W., R.F., N.B., and C.P. participated in data analysis and manuscript preparation. All authors discussed, read, and approved the final manuscript.

Funding: This work was financially supported by FONDEF ID15I10576, Proyecto Interno Multidisciplinario PIM_USM_12_18 (2018), Fondecyt Postdoctoral N°3160568 and Millennium Science Initiative P10-035F.

Conflicts of Interest: The authors declare no conflict of interest.

References

1. Flemming, H.C.; Wingender, J. The Biofilm Matrix. *Nat. Rev. Microbiol.* **2010**, *8*, 623–633. [CrossRef]
2. Simões, M.; Simoes, L.C.; Vieira, M.J. A Review of Current and Emergent Biofilm Control Strategies. *Food Sci. Technol.* **2010**, *43*, 573–583. [CrossRef]
3. Zhou, G.; Li, L.J.; Shi, Q.S.; Ouyang, Y.S.; Chen, Y.B.; Hu, W.F. Efficacy of Metal Ions and Isothiazolones in Inhibiting *Enterobacter cloacae* BF-17 Biofilm Formation. *Can. J. Microbiol.* **2013**, *60*, 5–14. [CrossRef] [PubMed]
4. Pal, A.; Paul, A.K. Optimization of Cultural Conditions for Production of Extracellular Polymeric Substances (EPS) by Serpentine rhizobacterium *Cupriavidus pauculus* KPS 201. *J. Polym.* **2013**, *2013*, 692374. [CrossRef]
5. Coenye, T.; Nelis, H.J. In Vitro and in Vivo Model Systems to Study Microbial Biofilm Formation. *J. Microbiol. Methods* **2010**, *83*, 89–105. [CrossRef] [PubMed]
6. Lee, J.H.; Choi, Y.K.; Kim, H.J.; Scheicher, R.H.; Cho, J.H. Physisorption of DNA nucleobases on h-BN and graphene: vdW-corrected DFT calculations. *J. Phys. Chem. C* **2013**, *117*, 13435–13441. [CrossRef]
7. McDougald, D.; Rice, S.A.; Barraud, N.; Steinberg, P.D.; Kjelleberg, S. Should We Stay or Should We Go: Mechanisms and Ecological Consequences for Biofilm Dispersal. *Nat. Rev. Microbiol.* **2011**, *10*, 39–50. [CrossRef] [PubMed]
8. Otter, J.A.; Vickery, K.; Walker, J.D.; deLancey Pulcini, E.; Stoodley, P.; Goldenberg, S.D.; Salkeld, J.A.; Chewins, J.; Yezli, S.; Edgeworth, J.D. Surface-attached Cells, Biofilms and Biocide Susceptibility: Implications for Hospital Cleaning and Disinfection. *J. Hosp. Infect.* **2015**, *89*, 16–27. [CrossRef] [PubMed]
9. De la Fuente-Núñez, C.; Reffuveille, F.; Fernández, L.; Hancock, R.E. Bacterial Biofilm Development as a Multicellular Adaptation: Antibiotic Resistance and New Therapeutic Strategies. *Curr. Opin. Microbiol.* **2013**, *16*, 580–589. [CrossRef]
10. Nyenje, M.E.; Green, E.; Ndip, R.N. Evaluation of the Effect of Different Growth Media and Temperature on the Suitability of Biofilm Formation by Enterobacter cloacae Strains Isolated from Food Samples in South Africa. *Molecules* **2013**, *18*, 9582–9593. [CrossRef]
11. Ciriminna, R.; Bright, F.V.; Pagliaro, M. Ecofriendly Antifouling Marine Coatings. *ACS Sustain. Chem. Eng.* **2015**, *3*, 559–565. [CrossRef]
12. Beściak, G.; Surmacz-Górska, J. Biofilm as a Basic Life Form of Bacteria. In Proceedings of the Polish-Swedish-Ukrainian Seminar, Krakow, Poland, 17–19 October 2011; pp. 1–8.
13. Brandes, J.; Kuhajek, J.M.; Goodwin, E.; Wood, S.A. Molecular Characterisation and Co-cultivation of Bacterial Biofilm Communities Associated with the Mat-Forming Diatom *Didymosphenia geminata*. *Microb. Ecol.* **2016**, *72*, 514–525. [CrossRef] [PubMed]
14. Ferreira, C.; Pereira, A.M.; Pereira, M.C.; Simões, M.; Melo, L.F. Biofilm Control with New Microparticles with Immobilized Biocide. *Heat Transf. Eng.* **2013**, *34*, 174–179. [CrossRef]
15. Ricart, M.; Guasch, H.; Alberch, M.; Barceló, D.; Bonnineau, C.; Geiszinger, A.; Ferrer, J.; Ricciardi, F.; Romaní, A.M.; Morin, S.; et al. Triclosan Persistence Through Wastewater Treatment Plants and Its Potential Toxic Effects on River Biofilms. *Aquat. Toxicol.* **2010**, *100*, 346–353. [CrossRef]
16. Zhang, C.; Cui, F.; Zeng, G.M.; Jiang, M.; Yang, Z.Z.; Yu, Z.G.; Zhu, M.Y.; Shen, L.Q. Quaternary Ammonium Compounds (QACs): A Review on Occurrence, Fate and Toxicity in The Environment. *Sci. Total. Environ.* **2015**, *518*, 352–362. [CrossRef]
17. Davison, W.M.; Pitts, B.; Stewart, P.S. Spatial and Temporal Patterns of Biocide Action against *Staphylococcus epidermidis* Biofilms. *Antimicrob. Agents Chemother.* **2010**, *54*, 2920–2927. [CrossRef]
18. Cos, P.; Tote, K.; Horemans, T.; Maes, L. Biofilms: An Extra Hurdle for Effective Antimicrobial Therapy. *Curr. Pharm. Des.* **2010**, *16*, 2279–2295. [CrossRef]
19. Cappitelli, F.; Polo, A.; Villa, F. Biofilm Formation in Food Processing Environments is Still Poorly Understood and Controlled. *Food Eng. Rev.* **2014**, *6*, 29–42. [CrossRef]
20. Musico, Y.L.; Santos, C.M.; Dalida, M.L.; Rodrigues, D.F. Surface modification of membrane filters using graphene and graphene oxide-based nanomaterials for bacterial inactivation and removal. *ACS Sustain. Chem. Eng.* **2014**, *2*, 1559–1565. [CrossRef]
21. Rizzello, L.; Cingolani, R.; Pompa, P.P. Nanotechnology Tools for Antibacterial Materials. *Nanomedicine* **2013**, *8*, 807–821. [CrossRef]
22. Rodrigues, D.F.; Elimelech, M. Toxic Effects of Single-walled Carbon Nanotubes in the Development of *E. coli* Biofilm. *Environ. Sci. Technol.* **2010**, *44*, 4583–4589. [CrossRef] [PubMed]

23. Hegab, H.M.; ElMekawy, A.; Zou, L.; Mulcahy, D.; Saint, C.P.; Ginic-Markovic, M. The Controversial Antibacterial Activity of Graphene-Based Materials. *Carbon* **2016**, *105*, 362–376. [CrossRef]
24. Chen, L.; Hu, P.; Zhang, L.; Huang, S.; Luo, L.; Huang, C. Toxicity of Graphene Oxide and Multi-walled Carbon Nanotubes Against Human Cells and Zebrafish. *Sci. China Chem.* **2012**, *55*, 2209–2216. [CrossRef]
25. Kalishwaralal, K.; BarathManiKanth, S.; Pandian, S.R.; Deepak, V.; Gurunathan, S. Silver Nanoparticles Impede the Biofilm Formation by *Pseudomonas aeruginosa* and *Staphylococcus epidermidis*. *Colloids Surf. B* **2010**, *79*, 340–344. [CrossRef] [PubMed]
26. Marambio-Jones, C.; Hoek, E.M. A review of the Antibacterial Effects of Silver Nanomaterials and Potential Implications for Human Health and the Environment. *J. Nanopart. Res.* **2010**, *12*, 1531–1551. [CrossRef]
27. Díez-Pascual, A.M. Antibacterial Activity of Nanomaterials. *Nanomaterials* **2018**, *8*, 359. [CrossRef] [PubMed]
28. Perreault, F.; Oukarroum, A.; Pirastru, L.; Sirois, L.; Gerson, M.W.; Popovic, R. Evaluation of Copper Oxide Nanoparticles Toxicity Using Chlorophyll Fluorescence Imaging in Lemna Gibba. *J. Bot.* **2010**, *2010*, 763142. [CrossRef]
29. Akhavan, O.; Ghaderi, E. Toxicity of Graphene and Graphene Oxide Nanowalls against Bacteria. *ACS Nano* **2010**, *4*, 5731–5736. [CrossRef]
30. Perreault, F.; De Faria, A.F.; Nejati, S.; Elimelech, M. Antimicrobial Properties of Graphene Oxide Nanosheets: Why Size Matters. *ACS Nano* **2015**, *9*, 7226–7236. [CrossRef] [PubMed]
31. Huang, X.; Liu, F.; Jiang, P.; Tanaka, T. Is Graphene Oxide an Insulating Material? In Proceedings of the 2013 IEEE International Conference on Solid Dielectrics (ICSD), Bologna, Italy, 30 June–4 July 2013; pp. 904–907.
32. Dreyer, D.R.; Park, S.; Bielawski, C.W.; Ruoff, R.S. The chemistry of graphene oxide. *Chem. Soc. Rev.* **2010**, *39*, 228–240. [CrossRef] [PubMed]
33. Parra, C.; Montero-Silva, F.; Henríquez, R.; Flores, M.; Garín, C.; Ramírez, C.; Moreno, M.; Correa, J.; Seeger, M.; Häberle, P. Suppressing Bacterial Interaction with Copper Surfaces Through Graphene and Hexagonal-boron Nitride Coatings. *ACS Appl. Mater. Interfaces* **2015**, *7*, 6430–6437. [CrossRef] [PubMed]
34. Parra, C.; Dorta, F.; Jimenez, E.; Henríquez, R.; Ramírez, C.; Rojas, R.; Villalobos, P. A Nanomolecular Approach to Decrease Adhesion of Biofouling-producing Bacteria to Graphene-coated Material. *J. Nanobiotechnol.* **2015**, *13*, 82. [CrossRef] [PubMed]
35. Wang, J.; Ma, F.; Sun, M. Graphene, Hexagonal Boron Nitride, and Their Heterostructures: Properties and Applications. *RSC Adv.* **2017**, *7*, 16801–16822. [CrossRef]
36. Parra, C.; Montero-Silva, F.; Gentil, D.; del Campo, V.; Henrique Rodrigues da Cunha, T.; Henríquez, R.; Häberle, P.; Garín, C.; Ramírez, C.; Fuentes, R.; et al. The Many Faces of Graphene as Protection Barrier. Performance under Microbial Corrosion and Ni Allergy Conditions. *Materials* **2017**, *10*, 1406. [CrossRef] [PubMed]
37. Song, L.; Ci, L.; Lu, H.; Sorokin, P.B.; Jin, C.; Ni, J.; Kvashnin, A.G.; Kvashnin, D.G.; Lou, J.; Yakobson, B.I.; et al. Large Scale Growth and Characterization of Atomic Hexagonal Boron Nitride Layers. *Nano Lett.* **2010**, *10*, 3209–3215. [CrossRef] [PubMed]
38. Shi, Y.; Hamsen, C.; Jia, X.; Kim, K.K.; Reina, A.; Hofmann, M.; Hsu, A.L.; Zhang, K.; Li, H.; Juang, Z.Y.; et al. Synthesis of Few-layer Hexagonal Boron Nitride Thin film by Chemical Vapor Deposition. *Nano Lett.* **2010**, *10*, 4134–4139. [CrossRef] [PubMed]
39. Mezzatesta, M.L.; Gona, F.; Stefani, S. Enterobacter cloacae Complex: Clinical Impact and Emerging Antibiotic Resistance. *Future Microbiol.* **2012**, *7*, 887–902. [CrossRef]
40. Bruinsma, G.M.; Van der Mei, H.C.; Busscher, H.J. Bacterial Adhesion to Surface Hydrophilic and Hydrophobic Contact Lenses. *Biomaterials* **2001**, *22*, 3217–3224. [CrossRef]
41. Ramírez, C.; Gallegos, I.; Ihl, M.; Bifani, V. Study of Contact Angle, Wettability and Water Vapor Permeability in Carboxymethylcellulose (CMC) Based Film with Murta Leaves (*Ugni molinae* Turcz) Extract. *J. Food Eng.* **2012**, *109*, 424–429. [CrossRef]
42. O'Toole, G.A. Microtiter Dish Biofilm Formation Assay. *J. Vis. Exp.* **2011**, *47*, 10–11. [CrossRef]
43. Nishijima, K.A.; Couey, H.M.; Alvarez, A.M. Internal yellowing, a bacterial disease of papaya fruits caused by Enterobacter cloacae. *Plant Dis.* **1987**, *71*, 1029–1034. [CrossRef]
44. Clarridge, J.E. Impact of 16S rRNA gene sequence analysis for identification of bacteria on clinical microbiology and infectious diseases. *Clin. Microbiol. Rev.* **2004**, *17*, 840–862. [CrossRef] [PubMed]
45. Chelius, M.K.; Triplett, E.W. The Diversity of Archaea and Bacteria in Association with The Roots of *Zea mays* L. *Microb. Ecol.* **2001**, *41*, 252–263. [CrossRef]

46. Rochelle, P.A.; Fry, J.C.; John Parkes, R.; Weightman, A.J. DNA Extraction for 16S rRNA Gene Analysis to Determine Genetic Diversity in Deep Sediment Communities. *FEMS Microbiol. Lett.* **1992**, *100*, 59–65. [CrossRef] [PubMed]
47. Bernstein, R.; Freger, V.; Lee, J.H.; Kim, Y.G.; Lee, J.; Herzberg, M. Should I Stay or Should I Go? Bacterial Attachment vs. Biofilm Formation on Surface-modified Membranes. *Biofouling* **2014**, *30*, 367–376. [CrossRef] [PubMed]
48. Longo, F.; Vuotto, C.; Donelli, G. Biofilm Formation in *Acinetobacter baumannii*. *New Microbiol.* **2014**, *37*, 119–127.
49. Zhao, Q.; Liu, Y.; Wang, C.; Wang, S.; Peng, N.; Jeynes, C. Bacterial Adhesion on Ion-implanted Stainless Steel Surfaces. *Appl. Surf. Sci.* **2007**, *253*, 8674–8681. [CrossRef]
50. Gao, L.; Pan, X.; Zhang, D.; Mu, S.; Lee, D.J.; Halik, U. Extracellular polymeric substances buffer against the biocidal effect of H_2O_2 on the bloom-forming cyanobacterium Microcystis aeruginosa. *Water Res.* **2015**, *1*, 51–58. [CrossRef]
51. Rayner, J.; Veeh, R.; Flood, J. Prevalence of microbial biofilms on selected fresh produce and household surfaces. *Int. J. Food Microbiol.* **2004**, *95*, 29–39. [CrossRef]
52. Merritt, J.H.; Kadouri, D.E.; O'Toole, G.A. Growing and Analyzing Static Biofilms. *Curr. Protoc. Microbiol.* **2011**, *22*. [CrossRef]
53. Huang, R.; Li, M.; Gregory, R.L. Bacterial Interactions in Dental Biofilm. *Virulence* **2011**, *2*, 435–444. [CrossRef] [PubMed]
54. Tegou, E.; Magana, M.; Katsogridaki, A.E.; Ioannidis, A.; Raptis, V.; Jordan, S.; Chatzipanagiotou, S.; Chatzandroulis, S.; Ornelas, C.; Tegos, G.P. Terms of Endearment: Bacteria Meet Graphene Nanosurfaces. *Biomaterials* **2016**, *89*, 38–55. [CrossRef] [PubMed]
55. Shellenberger, K.; Logan, B.E. Effect of Molecular Scale Roughness of Glass Beads on Colloidal and Bacterial Deposition. *Environ. Sci. Technol.* **2002**, *36*, 184–189. [CrossRef] [PubMed]
56. Li, B.; Logan, B.E. Bacterial Adhesion to Glass and Metal-oxide Surfaces. *Colloids Surf. B* **2004**, *36*, 81–90. [CrossRef] [PubMed]
57. Yankowitz, M.; Xue, J.; Cormode, D.; Sanchez-Yamagishi, J.D.; Watanabe, K.; Taniguchi, T.; Jarillo-Herrero, P.; Jacquod, P.; LeRoy, B.J. Emergence of Superlattice Dirac Points in Graphene on Hexagonal Boron Nitride. *Nat. Phys.* **2012**, *8*, 382. [CrossRef]
58. Liu, L.; Park, J.; Siegel, D.A.; McCarty, K.F.; Clark, K.W.; Deng, W.; Basile, L.; Idrobo, J.C.; Li, A.P.; Gu, G. Heteroepitaxial Growth of Two-dimensional Hexagonal Boron Nitride Templated by Graphene Edges. *Science* **2014**, *343*, 163–167. [CrossRef] [PubMed]
59. Ngo, T.T.; Le, D.Q.; Nguyen, X.N.; Phan, N.M. Synthesis of Multi-layer Graphene Films on Copper Tape by Atmospheric Pressure Chemical Vapor Deposition Method. *Adv. Nat. Sci. Nanosci. Nanotechnol.* **2013**, *4*, 035012.
60. Caneva, S.; Weatherup, R.S.; Bayer, B.C.; Blume, R.; Cabrero-Vilatela, A.; Braeuninger-Weimer, P.; Martin, M.B.; Wang, R.; Baehtz, C.; Schloegl, R.; et al. Controlling Catalyst Bulk Reservoir Effects for Monolayer Hexagonal Boron Nitride CVD. *Nano Lett.* **2016**, *16*, 1250–1261. [CrossRef]
61. Liu, N.; Pan, Z.; Fu, L.; Zhang, C.; Dai, B.; Liu, Z. The Origin of Wrinkles on Transferred Graphene. *Nano Res.* **2011**, *4*, 996. [CrossRef]
62. Li, J.; Wang, G.; Zhu, H.; Zhang, M.; Zheng, X.; Di, Z.; Liu, X.; Wang, X. Antibacterial Activity of Large-area Monolayer Graphene Film Manipulated by Charge Transfer. *Sci. Rep.* **2014**, *4*, 4359. [CrossRef]
63. Song, F.; Koo, H.; Ren, D. Effects of material properties on bacterial adhesion and biofilm formation. *J. Dent. Res.* **2015**, *94*, 1027–1034. [CrossRef] [PubMed]
64. Cerca, N.; Pier, G.B.; Vilanova, M.; Oliveira, R.; Azeredo, J. Quantitative Analysis of Adhesion and Biofilm Formation on Hydrophilic and Hydrophobic Surfaces of Clinical Isolates of *Staphylococcus epidermidis*. *Res. Microbiol.* **2005**, *156*, 506–514. [CrossRef] [PubMed]
65. Malanovic, N.; Lohner, K. Gram-positive Bacterial Cell Envelopes: The Impact on the Activity of Antimicrobial Peptides. *Biochim. Biophys. Acta* **2016**, *1858*, 936–946. [CrossRef] [PubMed]
66. Elimelech, M.; Gregory, J.; Jia, X. *Particle Deposition and Aggregation: Measurement, Modelling and Simulation*; Butterworth-Heinemann: Oxford, UK, 2013.
67. Itoh, H.; Sakuma, H. Dielectric Constant of Water as a Function of Separation in a Slab Geometry: A Molecular Dynamics Study. *J. Chem. Phys.* **2015**, *142*, 184703. [CrossRef] [PubMed]

68. Ducker, W.A.; Senden, T.J.; Pashley, R.M. Measurement of Forces in Liquids Using a Force Microscope. *Langmuir* **1992**, *8*, 1831–1836. [CrossRef]
69. Dupont-Gillain, C.C.; Nonckreman, C.J.; Adriaensen, Y.; Rouxhet, P.G. Fabrication of Surfaces with Bimodal Roughness through Polyelectrolyte/Colloid Assembly. In *Advances in Unconventional Lithography*; InTech: Vienna, Austria, 2011.
70. Deshpande, A.; Bao, W.; Miao, F.; Lau, C.N.; LeRoy, B.J. Spatially Resolved Spectroscopy of Monolayer Graphene on SiO_2. *Phys. Rev. B* **2009**, *79*, 205411. [CrossRef]
71. Lei, W.; Mochalin, V.N.; Liu, D.; Qin, S.; Gogotsi, Y.; Chen, Y. Boron Nitride Colloidal Solutions, Ultralight Aerogels and Freestanding Membranes Through One-step Exfoliation and Functionalization. *Nat. Commun.* **2015**, *6*, 8849. [CrossRef]
72. Van Merode, A.E.; Pothoven, D.C.; Van Der Mei, H.C.; Busscher, H.J.; Krom, B.P. Surface Charge Influences Enterococcal Prevalence in Mixed-species Biofilms. *J. Appl. Microbiol.* **2007**, *102*, 1254–1260. [CrossRef]
73. Busscher, H.J.; Weerkamp, A.H. Specific and Non-specific Interactions in Bacterial Adhesion to Solid Substrata. *FEMS Microbiol. Lett.* **1987**, *46*, 165–173. [CrossRef]
74. Kalin, M.; Polajnar, M. The Wetting of Steel, DLC Coatings, Ceramics and Polymers with Oils and Water: The Importance and Correlations of Surface Energy, Surface Tension, Contact Angle and Spreading. *Appl. Surf. Sci.* **2014**, *293*, 97–108. [CrossRef]

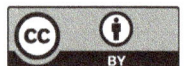

© 2019 by the authors. Licensee MDPI, Basel, Switzerland. This article is an open access article distributed under the terms and conditions of the Creative Commons Attribution (CC BY) license (http://creativecommons.org/licenses/by/4.0/).

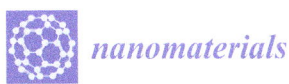

Article

Enhanced Photodynamic Anticancer Activities of Multifunctional Magnetic Nanoparticles (Fe$_3$O$_4$) Conjugated with Chlorin e6 and Folic Acid in Prostate and Breast Cancer Cells

Kyong-Hoon Choi [1], Ki Chang Nam [2], Guangsup Cho [3], Jin-Seung Jung [4,*] and Bong Joo Park [1,3,*]

1. Institute of Biomaterials, Kwangwoon University, Nowon-gu, Seoul 01897, Korea; solidchem@hanmail.net
2. Department of Medical Engineering, Dongguk University College of Medicine, Gyeonggi-do 10326, Korea; kichang.nam@gmail.com
3. Department of Electrical & Biological Physics, Kwangwoon University, Nowon-gu, Seoul 01897, Korea; gscho@kw.ac.kr
4. Department of Chemistry, Gangneung-Wonju National University, Gangneung 25457, Korea
* Correspondence: jjscm@gwnu.ac.kr (J.-S.J.); parkbj@kw.ac.kr (B.J.P.);
  Tel.: +82-33-640-2305 (J.-S.J.); +82-2-940-8629 (B.J.P.)

Received: 29 August 2018; Accepted: 12 September 2018; Published: 13 September 2018

Abstract: Photodynamic therapy (PDT) is a promising alternative to conventional cancer treatment methods. Nonetheless, improvement of in vivo light penetration and cancer cell-targeting efficiency remain major challenges in clinical photodynamic therapy. This study aimed to develop multifunctional magnetic nanoparticles conjugated with a photosensitizer (PS) and cancer-targeting molecules via a simple surface modification process for PDT. To selectively target cancer cells and PDT functionality, core magnetic (Fe$_3$O$_4$) nanoparticles were covalently bound with chlorin e6 (Ce6) as a PS and folic acid (FA). When irradiated with a 660-nm long-wavelength light source, the Fe$_3$O$_4$-Ce6-FA nanoparticles with good biocompatibility exerted marked anticancer effects via apoptosis, as confirmed by analyzing the translocation of the plasma membrane, nuclear fragmentation, activities of caspase-3/7 in prostate (PC-3) and breast (MCF-7) cancer cells. Ce6, used herein as a PS, is thus more useful for PDT because of its ability to produce a high singlet oxygen quantum yield, which is owed to deep penetration by virtue of its long-wavelength absorption band; however, further in vivo studies are required to verify its biological effects for clinical applications.

Keywords: multifunctional magnetic nanoparticles; chlorin e6; folic acid; in vivo penetration depth; cancer cell targeting

---

1. Introduction

Cancer is a leading cause of mortality worldwide. Every year, an estimated 11 million individuals are diagnosed with cancer, and approximately 7 million individuals die of cancer according to the World Health Organization (WHO) [1]. Therefore, cancer currently ranks among the deadliest diseases, and advancements in medical technology have yielded various methods for cancer treatment over the last few decades [2]. Among them, traditional chemotherapy is limited by its severe toxicity, poor tumor-specific delivery, and the possibility of inducing multi-drug resistance [3–5]. However, in comparison with chemotherapy, photodynamic therapy (PDT) offers certain unique advantages including minimal invasiveness, fewer side effects, negligible chemotherapeutic resistance, and low systematic toxicity [6–8].

In PDT, photosensitizers (PS) are the key components that transfer photo-energy to the surrounding O_2 molecules, generating reactive oxygen species (ROS), primarily singlet oxygen ($^1O_2$), to eliminate proximal cancer cells [9–12]. According to a recent study, various PSs have developed, which absorb light over a broad range from ultraviolet (UV) to the near-infrared (NIR) range [13,14]. However, the absorption bands of many PSs are primarily in the UV-Vis region [15,16]. Furthermore, the PSs with the absorption band in the NIR range have low $^1O_2$ quantum yield owing to a low population of PSs in the triplet state [17,18]. Therefore, these PSs are often limited by their low $^1O_2$ quantum yields, and low depth of penetration resulting from a short excitation wavelength [15,16]. In addition, currently available PSs are mostly nonspecifically activated and have poor water solubility and stability and low accumulation at the target site, resulting in treatment-related toxicity, light-induced degradation of drug molecules, and other side effects on adjacent normal tissue and blood cells [6,19–21]. To overcome these limitations, various inorganic and organic nanocarriers, including Fe_3O_4 nanoclusters, Au nanoparticles, graphene oxide, mesoporous silica nanoparticles, and polymer micelles, have been used to improve the stability and therapeutic outcomes of these PSs [22–26]. Nonetheless, the development of multifunctional nanoparticles with enhanced anticancer efficiency remains a major challenge in PDT.

Herein, to achieve enhanced photodynamic anticancer activity, we designed and fabricated a novel Fe_3O_4 nanoparticle conjugated with chlorin e6 (Ce6) and folic acid (FA) (Fe_3O_4-Ce6-FA) via simple surface modification. To enhance the PDT efficiency, magnetic core particles were conjugated with Ce6 and FA as PDT agents to increase the in vivo penetration depth of the light source and selectively eliminate cancer cells. In addition, we evaluated the efficiency of the Fe_3O_4-Ce6-FA nanoparticles for specific targeting and photodynamic anticancer activity in vitro. The Fe_3O_4-Ce6-FA nanoparticles developed herein could be a promising multifunctional nanoreagent for photodynamic tumor therapy and multifunctional drug delivery in the future.

2. Results and Discussion

2.1. Characterization of Multifunctional Fe_3O_4-Ce6-FA

Multifunctional 20-nm Fe_3O_4-Ce6-FA nanoparticles were fabricated via a simple surface modification via a wet chemical process as shown in Scheme 1. Ce6, having a long-wavelength absorption band and high singlet oxygen quantum yield, was conjugated with Fe ions on the surface of the Fe_3O_4 nanoparticles via esterification. Additionally, the multifunctional nanoparticles were functionalized with FA used as a targeting molecule to deliver these particles to the cancer cell membrane.

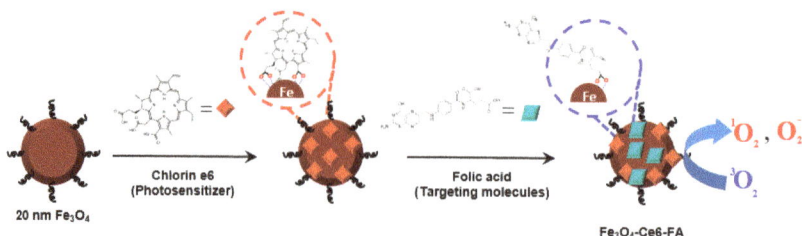

Scheme 1. Fabrication procedure for the multifunctional magnetic nanoparticles.

Transmission electron microscopy (TEM), field emission scanning electron microscopy (FE-SEM), and X-ray diffraction (XRD) analysis were performed to confirm the appearance, size distribution, and crystallinity of the Fe_3O_4-Ce6-FA nanoparticles. As shown in Figure 1a,b, Fe_3O_4-Ce6-FA nanoparticles had a uniform spherical structure and a rough surface, measuring approximately 20 nm in diameter (Figure 1a inset). High-resolution TEM (HRTEM) images revealed regular parallel lattice fringes, indicating the high crystallinity of the Fe_3O_4-Ce6-FA nanoparticles (inset of Figure 1b).

The lattice spacing of 0.26 nm was consistent with the in-plane lattice spacing of the (311) planes in the typical spinel structure of magnetite nanoparticles. The size histogram indicates that the average size of the particles was 19.8 nm with a distribution of 1.16 nm (Figure 1c). The wide-angle XRD pattern of Fe_3O_4-Ce6-FA nanoparticles can be indexed to the typical cubic structure of spinel Fe_3O_4 (JCPDS No. 19-629). The six strong Bragg reflection peaks (2θ = 30.2°, 35.7°, 43.4°, 53.6°, 57.4°, 63.0°), marked by their Miller indices ((220), (311), (400), (422), (511), and (440)) were obtained from standard Fe_3O_4 powder diffraction data (Figure 1d).

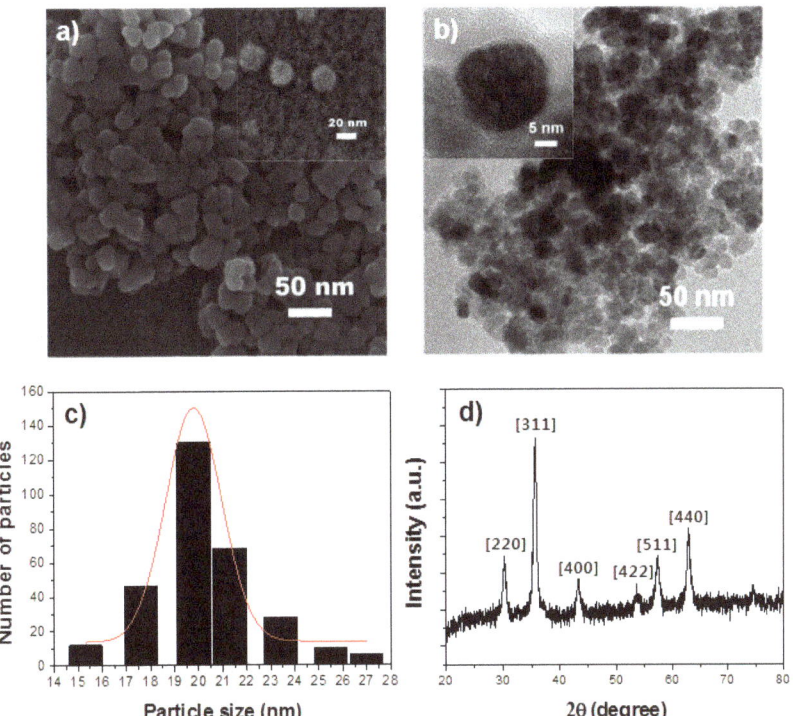

Figure 1. Structural analysis of the cholrin6- and folic acid-conjugated magnetite (Fe_3O_4-Ce6-FA) nanoparticles. (**a**) Field emission scanning electron and (**b**) transmission electron micrographs of the Fe_3O_4-Ce6-FA nanoparticles; (**c**) histogram of particle size distribution; (**d**) X-ray diffraction pattern of the Fe_3O_4-Ce6-FA nanoparticles.

Figure 2a shows the magnetic hysteresis loops of pure Fe_3O_4 and Fe_3O_4-Ce6-FA nanoparticles at room temperature. As shown, both samples exhibited superparamagnetic behavior without obvious remnant magnetization and coercivity owing to their small magnetite nanocrystal composition. The saturation magnetization (Ms) of pure Fe_3O_4 was 80.5 emu/g. After coating with PS and FA, the Ms of Fe_3O_4-Ce6-FA nanoparticles decreased to 58.5 emu/g. The minor reduction in magnetization primarily resulted from the reduction in the density of Fe_3O_4 due to the presence of non-magnetic coating layers. However, the Fe_3O_4-Ce6-FA nanoparticles (20 nm) still showed strong magnetization, thereby suggesting their suitability for magnetic separation and magnetic resonance (MR) imaging.

Figure 2b shows the photoluminescence (PL) and photoluminescence excitation (PLE) spectra of the pure Ce6 and the Fe_3O_4-Ce6-FA nanoparticles in THF. Ce6 displayed three main UV-Vis absorption peaks with an intense Soret band at 400 nm and two relatively weak Q-bands at 500 and 662 nm, respectively. After encapsulation of the Fe_3O_4 nanoparticles, a remarkable red shift and peak broadening in the UV-Vis spectrum of Fe_3O_4-Ce6-FA nanoparticles were observed, indicating the strong bonding between Ce6 and the magnetite nanoparticle [27]. Upon excitation at 660 nm, free Ce6 exhibited two strong emission peaks at 672 and 707 nm. The Fe_3O_4-Ce6-FA nanoparticles also exhibited a red shift and broadening compared with free Ce6, concurrent with the phenomenon observed during absorption.

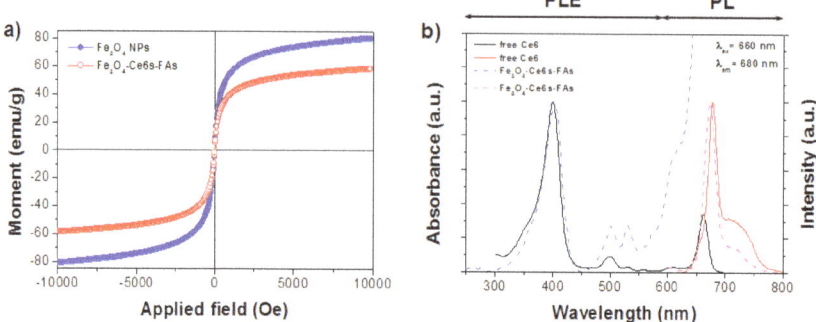

Figure 2. Magnetic and optical properties of the cholrin6- and folic acid-conjugated magnetite (Fe_3O_4-Ce6-FA) nanoparticles. (**a**) Room temperature magnetic hysteresis loops of pure Fe_3O_4 and Fe_3O_4-Ce6-FA nanoparticles; (**b**) Photoluminescence and photoluminescence excitation spectra of free Ce6 and the Fe_3O_4-Ce6-FA in THF.

We used 1,3-diphenylisobenzofuran (DPBF), a specific $^1O_2$ probe, to quantify the $^1O_2$ generated from the Fe_3O_4-Ce6-FA nanoparticles by monitoring the absorbance of DPBF at 424 nm. Figure 3a exhibits the time-dependent UV-Vis absorption spectra of complexes of DPBF and Fe_3O_4-Ce6-FA in ethanol, which were irradiated with a red light-emitting diode (LED) light source. Upon excitation at 660 nm, the intensity of the absorbance peak of DPBF at 424 nm decreased gradually with the increase in irradiation time in the presence of the Fe_3O_4-Ce6-FA nanoparticles (Figure 3b). In the blank condition, no appreciable degradation of DPBF was observed after irradiation for 35 min. Near-complete photodegradation of DPBF in the presence of Fe_3O_4-Ce6-FA nanoparticles was observed within 35 min. This clearly indicates that the Fe_3O_4-Ce6-FA nanoparticles can effectively generate the $^1O_2$ ROS. Based on the reaction kinetics, which was well fitted into the equation $\ln(C/C_0) = -k_{obs} \times \text{time (min)}$, the apparent first-order rate constant, k_{obs}, of DPBF photo-oxidation was 0.05094 min^{-1} for the Fe_3O_4-Ce6-FA nanoparticles (Figure 3c).

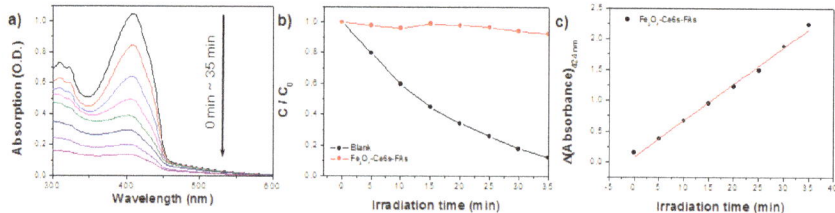

Figure 3. (**a**) UV-Vis spectra of 1,3-diphenylisobenzofuran (DPBF) in ethanol with the chlorin e6- and folic acid-conjugated magnetite (Fe_3O_4-Ce6-FA) nanoparticles in accordance with the irradiation time with a red LED lamp (λ_{max} = 660 nm); (**b**) The kinetic curve of the photodegradation efficiency of DPBF as a function of irradiation time; (**c**) Comparison of first-order degradation rates of DPBF.

2.2. In Vitro Cytotoxicity of Multifunctional Fe_3O_4-Ce6-FA Nanoparticles

For biomaterials to be used for biomedical applications, a basic biocompatibility assay is necessary to evaluate their cytotoxicity. Therefore, the in vitro cytotoxicity of Fe_3O_4-Ce6-FA was evaluated in normal fibroblast (L-929), breast cancer (MCF-7), and prostate cancer (PC-3) cell lines, as described previously [28–33]. Twofold-diluted concentrations of Fe$_3$O$_4$-Ce6-FA from 100 to 6.25 µg/mL were tested, and non-treated cells constituted the control. As shown in Figure 4a, the cell viabilities of all cells exceeded 95%, indicating that Fe$_3$O$_4$-Ce6-FA displayed no cytotoxicity in all cells, suggesting that Fe$_3$O$_4$-Ce6-FA nanoparticles may have biomedical applications with excellent biocompatibility.

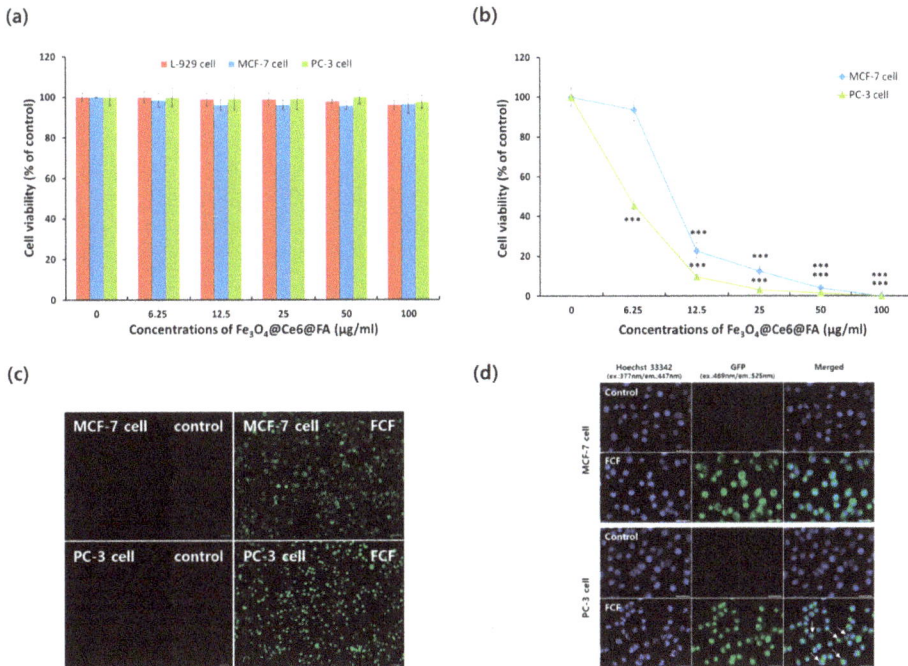

Figure 4. Biocompatibility and photodynamic anticancer activities of chlorin e6 and folic acid-conjugated magnetite (Fe$_3$O$_4$-Ce6-FA) nanoparticles. (**a**) Cytotoxicity and (**b**) phototoxicity of Fe$_3$O$_4$-Ce6-FA nanoparticles in MCF-7 (breast adenocarcinoma) and PC-3 (prostate adenocarcinoma) cell lines. Quantitative data are expressed as the mean ± standard deviation (n = 4), and the statistical comparisons were evaluated using Student's t-test. Significant differences were indicated by $p < 0.05$ (*** $p < 0.0005$ vs. control). (**c**) Images of MCF-7 and PC-3 cells after staining with fluorescein isothiocyanate-conjugated Annexin V (Annexin V-FITC) thus demonstrating the membrane translocation of the cells. The green fluorescence signal was produced by Annexin V-FITC. "FCF" represents Fe$_3$O$_4$-Ce6-FA nanoparticles. Scale bar = 50 µm. (**d**) Nuclear fragmentation and caspase-3/7 activity in MCF-7 and PC-3 cells. The cells were stained with Hoechst 33342 to detect nuclear fragmentation and CellEvent Caspase-3/7 Green Detection reagent to detect caspase-3/7 activity after 6 h post photodynamic therapy at 20 mW for 30 min. Arrows represent apoptotic bodies of cells. Scale bar= 30 µm.

2.3. In Vitro Photodynamic Anticancer Activity of Fe$_3$O$_4$-Ce6-FA Nanoparticles

To confirm the photo-killing ability of Fe$_3$O$_4$-Ce6-FA nanoparticles, PC-3 and MCF-7 cell lines were exposed to LED irradiation for 10 min after incubation with various concentrations of Fe$_3$O$_4$-Ce6-FA nanoparticles for 2 h. As shown in Figure 4b, cell viabilities of the two cell lines were significantly decreased with an increase in nanoparticle concentration, and the cell viability of PC-3 cells was even more drastically decreased compared to that of MCF-7 cells, even at the lowest concentration of 6.25 µg/mL. This indicated that the photo-killing efficacy of Fe$_3$O$_4$-Ce6-FA nanoparticles was concentration-dependent. Moreover, Fe$_3$O$_4$-Ce6-FA nanoparticles are more effective than Fe$_3$O$_4$ conjugated with hematoporphyrins (HPs) and FA, as reported previously [30,31]. The PS (Ce6) used herein is more applicable for PDT owing to its attributes, which include a high singlet oxygen quantum yield and long-wavelength absorption band, resulting in deeper light penetration in vivo compared with HP-conjugated nanoparticles. In other words, the photodynamic anticancer efficacy of Fe_3O_4-Ce6-FA nanoparticles was closely associated with singlet oxygen quantum yield and the concentration of the Fe_3O_4-Ce6-FA nanoparticles.

Considering the photodynamic anticancer activity of Fe_3O_4-Ce6-FA nanoparticles, the mechanisms underlying cancer cell death were evaluated via analysis of the translocation of the plasma membrane, using an Annexin V-fluorescein isothiocyanate (FITC) apoptosis detection kit, nuclear fragmentation using a fluorescent dye (Hoechst 33342), and enzyme activities of caspase-3/7 using a CellEvent Caspase-3/7 Green Detection reagent. First, PC-3 and MCF-7 cells were stained with Annexin V-FITC reagent post-irradiation after incubation with Fe_3O_4-Ce6-FA nanoparticles for 2 h to confirm phosphatidylserine translocation from the intracellular to the extracellular leaflet of the plasma membrane, which is a hallmark of the early stage of apoptotic cell death. Figure 4c shows the images of live and apoptotic cells stained with Annexin V-FITC, post-irradiation. Both cell types (MCF-7 and PC-3) in the Fe_3O_4-Ce6-FA nanoparticle-treated groups showed green fluorescence, whereas control cells did not. These results indicate that PDT following treatment with Fe_3O_4-Ce6-FA nanoparticles induced cancer cell death via apoptosis.

Additionally, nuclear fragmentation of cancer cells, which is also a hallmark of apoptotic cell death, was confirmed via staining with Hoechst 33342 dye. As shown in Figure 4d, the nuclei of both cell types treated with Fe_3O_4-Ce6-FA nanoparticles were more condensed than those of control cells, and most nuclei of PC-3 cells rapidly changed to granular apoptotic nuclear bodies. However, no changes were detected in the control cells of both cell lines. These results also indicated that irradiation after treatment with Fe_3O_4-Ce6-FA nanoparticles enhanced apoptotic cell death.

Finally, caspase-3/7 activity, which essentially contributes to apoptotic cell death, were also evaluated using a fluorogenic substrate highly specific for activated caspase-3 and -7. As shown in Figure 4d, both cell types (MCF-7 and PC-3) treated with Fe_3O_4-Ce6-FA nanoparticles showed strong green fluorescence. Moreover, the PC-3 cells treated with Fe_3O_4-Ce6-FA nanoparticles showed morphological changes following irradiation, as indicated by the presence of apoptotic cellular bodies. These results indicate that cells treated with Fe_3O_4-Ce6-FA nanoparticles expressed high amounts of activated caspase-3 and -7 upon irradiation, and that the cells underwent apoptotic cell death. Overall, the results indicate that Fe_3O_4-Ce6-FA nanoparticles induced apoptotic cell death.

3. Materials and Methods

3.1. Preparation of Fe_3O_4-Ce6-FA Nanoparticles

Multifunctional Fe_3O_4-Ce6-FA nanocomposites were synthesized in accordance with a previously reported procedure with minor modifications [28]. In brief, $FeCl_3 \cdot 6H_2O$ (0.54 g) and $NaAc \cdot 3H_2O$ (1.5 g) in 20 mL ethylene glycol (EG) and diethylene glycol (DEG) (1:19) were added in a 200 mL round-bottom flask, and the mixture was vigorously stirred for 30 min. Thereafter, the yellowish homogeneous solution formed was sealed in a teflon-lined stainless steel autoclave. The autoclave was heated to and maintained at 200 °C for 10 h and cooled to ambient temperature. The black precipitate was harvested via magnetic decantation, washed with deionized water and absolute alcohol several times, and then dried in a vacuum oven at 60 °C for 12 h. The photoactive and targeting functionalities of the Fe_3O_4 nanoparticles were achieved using a wet chemical process similar to our previous method [29]. Briefly, 20 mg of precipitated Fe_3O_4 nanoparticles with 20 nm size were mixed with a solution of Ce6/EtOH (final concentration, 10^{-4} M). The Ce6 molecules are easily conjugated to the surface of magnetite nanoparticles owing to the three terminal carboxyl groups, which initiate covalent bonding. Furthermore, the Ce6 molecules have a high singlet oxygen quantum yield of 0.77 in solution [34]. This value of singlet oxygen quantum yield is higher than that of the other photosensitizers such as hematoporphyrin (0.51) [35] and protoporphyrin (0.63) [36]. The solution was vigorously agitated for 24 h at room temperature. After the reaction was completed, the product was washed several times with EtOH. To facilitate targeting functionality, the FA molecules were conjugated to Ce6-bonded Fe_3O_4 nanoparticles (Fe_3O_4-Ce6). Similarly, the washed Fe_3O_4-Ce6 nanoparticles were fully dispersed in 20 mL of FA/dimethylsulfoxide (DMSO) solution (3.7×10^{-4} M). The mixture solution was stirred for another 5 h at 25 °C. The Fe_3O_4-Ce6-FA nanocomposites were separated via magnetic decantation and washed with DMSO and phosphate-buffered saline (PBS; pH = 7.2) several times. Thereafter, the resulting nanoparticles were finally dried in vacuum at room temperature for 24 h. The concentration of HP and FA bonded to the surfaces of the Fe_3O_4 nanoparticles was estimated using UV-Vis absorption spectroscopy.

3.2. Physical Characterization of Multifunctional Fe_3O_4-Ce6-FA Particles

TEM (JEM-2100F, JEOL, Tokyo, Japan) and FE-SEM (SU-70, Hitachi, Tokyo, Japan) were performed to study the morphology of the multifunctional nanoparticles. The crystallographic structure of the composite particles was investigated via XRD (X'Pert Pro MPD, PANalytical, Almelo, Netherlands), using Cu Kα radiation. A vibrating sample magnetometer (VSM; Lakeshore 7300, Lake Shore Cryotronics, Westerville, OH, USA) was used to obtain magnetization versus magnetic field loop up to H = 10 kOe at room temperature. Steady-state absorption and PL and PLE spectra were measured using a UV–Vis spectrophotometer (U-2800, Hitachi, Tokyo, Japan) and spectrofluorometer (F-4500, Hitachi, Tokyo, Japan), respectively.

3.3. Biocompatibility of Fe_3O_4-Ce6-FA Nanoparticles

Cytotoxicity of the Fe_3O_4-Ce6-FA (FCF) nanoparticles was evaluated in L-929 (mouse fibroblasts), MCF-7 (breast adenocarcinoma), and PC-3 (prostate adenocarcinoma) cell lines, as described previously [28–33]. Briefly, all cells were seeded in a 24-well plate at 1.5×10^5 cells/mL and incubated at 37 °C in 5% CO_2 for 24 h, followed by further incubation with various concentrations (0, 6.25, 12.5, 25, 50, and 100 µg/mL) of FCF nanoparticles after exchanging the media with fresh media, in the dark. After another 24 h incubation, the viable cells were quantified using Cell Counting Kit-8 (CCK-8; Dojindo Laboratories, Kumamoto, Japan) assay reagent in accordance with the manufacturer's instructions after washing three times with Dulbecco's phosphate-buffered saline (DPBS). The optical density for each well was measured using a multimode microplate reader (Cytation 3, BioTek Instruments, Inc., Winooski, VT, USA) with an optical filter at 450 nm, and cell viability was determined in comparison with the untreated control.

3.4. Photodynamic Anticancer Activity of Multifunctional FCF Nanoparticles

Anticancer activity of the FCF nanoparticles was also assessed in MCF-7 and PC-3 cells on the basis of cell viability determined using CCK-8 after irradiation, as described previously [33–36]. Each cell type was plated in a 24-well plate at the same concentration and incubated as described in 3.3. Thereafter, the cells were further incubated with various concentrations (0, 6.25, 12.5, 25, 50, and 100 µg/mL) of FCF nanoparticles for 2 h in the dark, followed by three washes with DPBS, replenishment of the media, and irradiation with a red light-emitting diode (LED; FD-332R-N1, Fedy Technology Co., Shenzhen, China). The LEDs were driven using a constant current buck driver (LED-2800, TMC Co., Gunpo, Korea) and light intensity was regulated via pulse width modulation (CB210, Comfile Technology, Seoul, Korea). LED irradiation was applied at a maximum wavelength of 660 nm at 20 mW/cm^2. After irradiation for 30 min, cancer cells were further incubated for 24 h, and cell viability was determined via a CCK-8 assay, as described in Section 3.3.

To evaluate the mechanisms underlying cancer cell death by Fe_3O_4-Ce6-FA after irradiation, both cancer cell types pre-cultured for 24 h were further incubated with 12.5 µg/mL of FCF after replenishing media in the dark. After 2 h of incubation, each cell type was irradiated with LED light at the same power for 10 min, as described previously in this section, and further incubated for 6 h to induce cell death. Thereafter, the plasma membranes and nuclei of both cell types were stained with an Annexin V-FITC apoptosis detection reagent (Komabiotech Inc., Seoul, Korea), Hoechst 33342 dye (Invitrogen, Molecular Probes, Eugene, OR, USA), and a CellEvent Caspase-3/7 Green Detection reagent (Invitrogen) in accordance with the manufacturers' instructions. After staining each sample, fluorescence microscopic images were acquired using an automated live cell imager (Lionheart FX; BioTek Instruments, Inc., VT, USA).

4. Conclusions

In summary, we synthesized Fe_3O_4-Ce6-FA nanoparticles for FA receptor-targeted PDT. PS and FA were covalently bound to the surface of the magnetite nanoparticles. The prepared multifunctional Fe_3O_4-Ce6-FA nanocomposites had high water solubility and good biocompatibility without any cytotoxicity. Moreover, Fe_3O_4-Ce6-FA exhibited more effective anticancer activity via apoptosis in prostate (PC-3) and breast cancer (MCF-7) cell lines in comparison with Fe_3O_4 conjugated with HPs. Thus, the PS (Ce6) used in this study is more useful for PDT applications owing to its ability to produce a high singlet oxygen quantum yield and deep penetration owing to its long-wavelength absorption band. However, further in vivo studies are required to verify its biological effects for clinical applications, although we believe that our study makes a significant contribution to PDT because it supports the use of chlorin e6 as a PS in multifunctional nanomaterials for effective PTD.

Author Contributions: The manuscript was written through contribution of all authors. K.-H.C. and K.C.N. designed the experiments, performed it, and drafted the manuscript. G.C. helped to interpret the characterization data and wrote the manuscript. J.-S.J. and B.J.P conceived of the study, participated in its design and coordination, and helped to draft and review the manuscript. All authors have given approval to the final version of the manuscript. K.-H.C. and K.C.N. contributed equally to this work.

Funding: This study was supported financially by the Bio & Medical Technology Development Program of the National Research Foundation (NRF) funded by the Ministry of Science & ICT (grant numbers NRF-2015M3A9E2066855 and -2015M3A9E2066856) and by the Research Grant from Kwangwoon University in 2018. J.-S.J. thanks the National Research Foundation of Korea (NRF 2017R1D1A3B03027857) for financial support.

Conflicts of Interest: The authors declare no conflict of interest.

Abbreviations

CCK-8	Cell Counting Kit-8
Ce6	Chlorin e6
DPBF	1,3-Diphenylisobenzofuran
DPBS	Dulbecco's phosphate-buffered saline
FA	Folic acid
FCF	Fe_3O_4-Ce6-FA
FE-SEM	Field emission scanning electron microscopy
FITC	Fluorescein isothiocyanate
HPs	Hematoporphyrins
LED	Light-emitting diode
Ms	Saturation magnetization
PDT	Photodynamic therapy
PL	Photoluminescence
PLE	Photoluminescence excitation
PS	Photosensitizer
ROS	Reactive oxygen species
TEM	Transmission electron microscopy
XRD	X-ray diffraction

References

1. Ferlay, J.; Soerjomataram, I.; Dikshit, R.; Eser, S.; Mathers, C.; Rebelo, M.; Parkin, D.M.; Forman, D.; Bray, F. Cancer incidence and mortality worldwide: Sources, methods and major patterns in GLOBOCAN 2012. *Int. J. Cancer* **2015**, *136*, E359. [CrossRef] [PubMed]
2. Wang, Y.; Shim, M.S.; Levinson, N.S.; Sung, H.-W.; Xia, Y. Stimuli-responsive materials for controlled release of theranostic agents. *Adv. Funct. Mater.* **2014**, *24*, 4206–4220. [CrossRef] [PubMed]
3. Tian, G.; Zheng, X.; Zhang, X.; Yin, W.; Yu, J.; Wang, D.; Zhang, Z.; Yang, X.; Gu, Z.; Zhao, Y. TPGS-stabilized NaYbF$_4$: Er upconversion nanoparticles for dual-modal fluorescent/CT imaging and anticancer drug delivery to overcome multi-drug resistance. *Biomaterials* **2015**, *40*, 107–116. [CrossRef] [PubMed]
4. Patel, N.R.; Pattni, B.S.; Abouzeid, A.H.; Torchilin, V.P. Nanopreparations to overcome multidrug resistance in cancer. *Adv. Drug Deliv. Rev.* **2013**, *65*, 1748–1762. [CrossRef] [PubMed]
5. Song, G.; Wang, Q.; Wang, Y.; Lv, G.; Li, C.; Zou, R.; Chen, Z.; Qin, Z.; Huo, K.; Hu, R.; et al. A low-toxic multifunctional nanoplatform based on Cu$_9$S$_5$@mSiO$_2$ core-shell nanocomposites: Combining photothermal- and chemotherapies with infrared thermal imaging for cancer treatment. *Adv. Funct. Mater.* **2013**, *23*, 4281–4292. [CrossRef]
6. Lovell, J.F.; Liu, T.W.B.; Chen, J.; Zheng, G. Activatable photosensitizers for imaging and therapy. *Chem. Rev.* **2010**, *110*, 2839–2857. [CrossRef] [PubMed]
7. Celli, J.P.; Spring, B.Q.; Rizvi, I.; Evans, C.L.; Samkoe, K.S.; Verma, S.; Pogue, B.W.; Hasan, T. Imaging and photodynamic therapy: Mechanisms, monitoring, and optimization. *Chem. Rev.* **2010**, *110*, 2795–2838. [CrossRef] [PubMed]
8. Dolmans, D.E.; Fukumura, D.; Jain, R.K. Photodynamic therapy for cancer. *Nat. Rev. Cancer* **2003**, *3*, 380–387. [CrossRef]
9. Ding, X.; Han, B.H. Metallophthalocyanine-based conjugated microporous polymers as highly efficient photosensitizers for singlet oxygen generation. *Angew. Chem. Int. Ed.* **2015**, *54*, 6536–6539. [CrossRef] [PubMed]
10. Gong, H.; Dong, Z.; Liu, Y.; Yin, S.; Cheng, L.; Xi, W.; Xiang, J.; Liu, K.; Li, Y.; Liu, Z. Engineering of multifunctional nano-micelles for combined photothermal and photodynamic therapy under the guidance of multimodal imaging. *Adv. Funct. Mater.* **2014**, *24*, 6492–6502. [CrossRef]
11. Cakmak, Y.; Kolemen, S.; Duman, S.; Dede, Y.; Dolen, Y.; Kilic, B.; Kostereli, Z.; Yildirim, L.T.; Dogan, A.L.; Guc, D.; et al. Designing excited states: Theory-guided access to efficient photosensitizers for photodynamic action. *Angew. Chem. Int. Ed.* **2011**, *50*, 11937–11941. [CrossRef] [PubMed]
12. Agostinis, P.; Berg, K.; Cengel, K.A.; Foster, T.H.; Girotti, A.W.; Gollnick, S.O. Photodynamic therapy of cancer: An update. *CA Cancer J. Clin.* **2011**, *61*, 250–281. [CrossRef] [PubMed]
13. Luo, T.; Zhang, Q.; Lu, Q.-B. Photodynamic therapy mediated by indocyanine green with etoposide to treat non-small-cell lung cancer. *Cancer* **2017**, *9*, 63. [CrossRef] [PubMed]
14. Mou, J.; Lin, T.; Huang, F.; Shi, J.; Chen, H. A new green titania with enhanced NIR absorption for mitochondria-targeted cancer therapy. *Theranostics* **2017**, *7*, 1531–1542. [CrossRef] [PubMed]
15. Ge, J.; Lan, M.; Zhou, B.; Liu, W.; Guo, L.; Wang, H.; Jia, Q.; Niu, G.; Huang, X.; Zhou, H.; et al. A graphene quantum dot potodynamic therapy agent with high singlet oxygen generation. *Nat. Commun.* **2014**, *5*, 4596. [CrossRef] [PubMed]
16. Yogo, T.; Urano, Y.; Ishitsuka, Y.; Maniwa, F.; Nagano, T. Highly efficient and photostable photosensitizer based on bodipy chromophore. *J. Am. Chem. Soc.* **2005**, *127*, 12162–12163. [CrossRef] [PubMed]
17. Reindl, S.; Penzkofer, A.; Gong, S.-H.; Landthaler, M.; Szeimies, R.M.; Abels, C.; Bäumler, W. Quantum yield of triplet formation for indocyanine green. *J. Photochem. Photobiol. A* **1997**, *105*, 65–68. [CrossRef]
18. Tang, C.-Y.; Wu, F.-Y.; Yang, M.-K.; Guo, Y.-M.; Lu, G.-H.; Yang, Y.-H. A classic near-infrared probe indocyanine green for detecting singlet oxygen. *Int. J. Mol. Sci.* **2016**, *17*, 219. [CrossRef] [PubMed]
19. Zhen, Z.; Tang, W.; Chuang, Y.J.; Todd, T.; Zhang, W.; Lin, X. Tumor vasculature targeted photodynamic therapy for enhanced delivery of nanoparticles. *ACS Nano* **2014**, *8*, 6004–6013. [CrossRef] [PubMed]
20. Bechet, D.; Couleaud, P.; Frochot, C.; Viriot, M.; Guillemin, F.; Barberi-Heyob, M. Nanoparticles as vehicles for delivery of photodynamic therapy agents. *Trends Biotechnol.* **2008**, *26*, 612–621. [CrossRef] [PubMed]

21. Richter, A.M.; Waterfield, E.; Jain, A.K.; Canaan, A.J.; Allison, B.A.; Levy, J.G. Liposomal delivery of a photosensitizer, benzoporphyrin derivative monoacid ring A (BPD), to tumor tissue in a mouse tumor model. *Photochem. Photobiol.* **1993**, *57*, 1000–1006. [CrossRef] [PubMed]
22. Wang, C.; Xu, H.; Liang, C.; Liu, Y.; Li, Z.; Yang, G.; Cheng, H.; Li, Y.; Liu, Z. Iron oxide @ polypyrrole nanoparticles as a multifunctional drug carrier for remotely controlled cancer therapy with synergistic antitumor effect. *ACS Nano* **2013**, *7*, 6782–6795. [CrossRef] [PubMed]
23. Wang, Z.; Chen, Z.; Liu, Z.; Shi, P.; Dong, K.; Ju, E.; Ren, J.; Qu, X. A multi-stimuli responsive gold nanocage-hyaluronic platform for targeted photothermal and chemotherapy. *Biomaterials* **2014**, *35*, 9678–9688. [CrossRef] [PubMed]
24. Wang, Y.; Wang, K.; Zhao, J.; Liu, X.; Bu, J.; Yan, X.; Huang, R. Multifunctional mesoporous silica-coated graphene nanosheet used for chemo-photothermal synergistic targeted therapy of glioma. *J. Am. Chem. Soc.* **2013**, *135*, 4799–4804. [CrossRef] [PubMed]
25. Zhang, C.; Zhao, K.; Bu, W.; Ni, D.; Liu, Y.; Feng, J.; Shi, J. Marriage of scintillator and semiconductor for synchronous radiotherapy and deep photodynamic therapy with diminished oxygen dependence. *Angew. Chem. Int. Ed.* **2015**, *127*, 1790–1794. [CrossRef]
26. Elsabahy, M.; Heo, G.S.; Lim, S.-M.; Sun, G.; Wooley, K.L. Polymeric nanostructures for imaging and therapy. *Chem. Rev.* **2015**, *115*, 10967–11011. [CrossRef] [PubMed]
27. Choi, K.-H.; Wang, K.-K.; Oh, S.-L.; Im, J.-E.; Kim, B.-J.; Park, J.-C.; Choi, D.; Kim, H.-K.; Kim, Y.-R. Singlet oxygen generating nanolayer coatings on NiTi alloy for photodynamic application. *Surf. Coat. Technol.* **2010**, *205*, S62–S67. [CrossRef]
28. Choi, K.-H.; Nam, K.C.; Kim, U.-H.; Cho, G.; Jung, J.-S.; Park, B.J. Optimized photodynamic therapy with multifunctional cobalt magnetic nanoparticles. *Nanomaterials* **2017**, *7*, 144. [CrossRef] [PubMed]
29. Choi, K.-H.; Nam, K.C.; Malkinski, L.; Choi, E.H.; Jung, J.-S.; Park, B.J. Size-dependent photodynamic anticancer activity of biocompatible multifunctional magnetic submicron particles in prostate cancer cells. *Molecules* **2016**, *21*, 1187. [CrossRef] [PubMed]
30. Nam, K.C.; Choi, K.-H.; Lee, K.-D.; Kim, J.H.; Jung, J.-S.; Park, B.J. Particle size dependent photodynamic anticancer activity of hematoporphyrin-conjugated Fe_3O_4 particles. *J. Nanomater.* **2016**, *2016*, 1278393. [CrossRef]
31. Choi, K.H.; Nam, K.C.; Kim, H.J.; Min, J.; Uhm, H.S.; Choi, E.H.; Park, B.J. Synthesis and characterization of photo-functional magnetic nanoparticles (Fe_3O_4@HP) for applications in photodynamic cancer therapy. *J. Korean Phys. Soc.* **2014**, *65*, 1658–1662. [CrossRef]
32. Park, B.J.; Choi, K.H.; Nam, K.C.; Ali, A.; Min, J.E.; Son, H.; Uhm, H.S.; Kim, H.J.; Jung, J.S.; Choi, E.H. Photodynamic anticancer activities of multifunctional cobalt ferrite nanoparticles in various cancer cells. *J. Biomed. Nanotechnol.* **2015**, *11*, 226–235. [CrossRef] [PubMed]
33. Choi, K.H.; Choi, E.W.; Min, J.E.; Son, H.; Uhm, H.S.; Choi, E.H.; Park, B.J.; Jung, J.S. Comparison study on photodynamic anticancer activity of multifunctional magnetic particles by formation of cations. *IEEE Trans. Magn.* **2014**, *50*, 5200704. [CrossRef]
34. Paul, S.; Heng, W.S.; Chan, L.W. Optimization in solvent selection for chlorin e6 in photodynamic therapy. *J. Fluoresc.* **2013**, *23*, 283–291. [CrossRef] [PubMed]
35. Mathai, S.; Smith, T.A.; Ghiggino, K.P. Singlet oxygen quantum yields of potential porphyrin-based photosensitisers for photodynamic therapy. *Photochem. Photobiol. Sci.* **2007**, *6*, 995–1002. [CrossRef] [PubMed]
36. Rossi, L.M.; Silva, P.R.; Vono, L.L.R.; Fernandes, A.U.; Tada, D.B.; Baptista, M.S. Protoporphyrin IX nanoparticle carrier: Preparation, optical properties, and singlet oxygen generation. *Langmuir* **2008**, *24*, 12534–12538. [CrossRef] [PubMed]

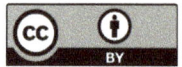

© 2018 by the authors. Licensee MDPI, Basel, Switzerland. This article is an open access article distributed under the terms and conditions of the Creative Commons Attribution (CC BY) license (http://creativecommons.org/licenses/by/4.0/).

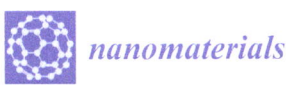

Article

A Comprehensive Cheminformatics Analysis of Structural Features Affecting the Binding Activity of Fullerene Derivatives

Natalja Fjodorova [1,*], Marjana Novič [1], Katja Venko [1] and Bakhtiyor Rasulev [2]

[1] National Institute of Chemistry, SI-1000 Ljubljana, Slovenia; marjana.novic@ki.si (M.N.); katja.venko@ki.si (K.V.)
[2] Department of Coatings and Polymeric Materials, North Dakota State University, Fargo, ND 58102, USA; bakhtiyor.rasulev@ndsu.edu
* Correspondence: natalja.fjodorova@ki.si

Received: 12 December 2019; Accepted: 27 December 2019; Published: 2 January 2020

Abstract: Nanostructures like fullerene derivatives (FDs) belong to a new family of nano-sized organic compounds. Fullerenes have found a widespread application in material science, pharmaceutical, biomedical, and medical fields. This fact caused the importance of the study of pharmacological as well as toxicological properties of this relatively new family of chemicals. In this work, a large set of 169 FDs and their binding activity to 1117 disease-related proteins was investigated. The structure-based descriptors widely used in drug design (so-called drug-like descriptors) were applied to understand cheminformatics characteristics related to the binding activity of fullerene nanostructures. Investigation of applied descriptors demonstrated that polarizability, topological diameter, and rotatable bonds play the most significant role in the binding activity of FDs. Various cheminformatics methods, including the counter propagation artificial neural network (CPANN) and Kohonen network as visualization tool, were applied. The results of this study can be applied to compose the priority list for testing in risk assessment related to the toxicological properties of FDs. The pharmacologist can filter the data from the heat map to view all possible side effects for selected FDs.

Keywords: fullerene derivatives; drug-like descriptors; binding activity; cheminformatics; neural networks modelling; hydrogenation; pharmacology; toxicology

---

1. Introduction

Fullerene derivatives (FDs) are a relatively new class of organic compounds belonging to nano-sized materials. These materials have opened up new opportunities in nanotechnology, as well as in medicine [1].

Fullerenes are commonly classified as "radical sponges" [2] due to their remarkable reactivity with free radicals [3–6]. The radical scavenging properties of fullerenes have found many applications in biological systems. They were applied for treatment of various free radical-induced biological disorders, including mostly neurodegenerative diseases (i.e., amyotrophic lateral sclerosis, Alzheimer's disease, Parkinson's disease) and other cytotoxic processes caused by oxidative stress. The fullerenes have found the application as cytoprotective agents against oxidative stress [7]. The FDs can prevent apoptosis by neutralization of reactive oxygen species (ROS). The antimicrobial property of FDs was demonstrated in [8] where authors showed the inhibition of *Escherichia coli* bacteria growth by FDs. The ability of fullerenes to fit inside the hydrophobic cavity of HIV proteases makes them a potentially good inhibitor of the catalytic active site of enzyme. Therefore, FDs have found their application as antiviral drugs [9–14]. The antiviral activity of FDs was found to be due to the antioxidant activity of them. At the same time, when fullerenes are exposed to a light, they can initiate formation of ROSs (singlet oxygen and superoxide), which leads to antibacterial/antimicrobial activity, and this effect of FDs is used in water treatment systems [11,15–19].

FD nanostructures can be used in many applications. The details about synthesis, chemistry, and application of fullerenes were reported in several reviews [6,20,21]. Toxicological studies of fullerenes were reported in [22]. Thus, pristine fullerenes have shown a low toxicity. At the same time, there is still a lack of knowledge related to toxicity of FDs per se.

Nanoparticles, including fullerenes, often pose a serious threat to human health, the environment, or both. Nanoparticles can cause toxic effects at different levels: Cellular, subcellular, and bio molecular [23,24]. In this regard, FDs also can have a significant impact on environment and human health and; therefore, these nanostructures need to be investigated as well for potential toxicological and environmental risk.

There is still a lack of knowledge about toxicity of FD nanostructures and their mechanisms of action in living organisms. To tackle this problem the research related to activity/safety of this class of chemicals is initiated in this work.

The novel approaches for risk assessment of nanomaterials using computational tools, like quantitative structure activity relationships (QSARs), are discussed in several publications [25–32]. Thus, reliable QSAR models can offer a time-effective and cost-effective measure of chemicals' properties in the absence of new experimental data. As per FDs, there are a number of computational studies and the application of cheminformatics tools including QSAR models for modelling and prediction of FDs' properties, including HIV protease inhibition, which is also discussed in articles [33–35].

In last years, the risk assessment of chemicals has focused on the mechanistic interpretation of QSAR models based on description of the relationship between the descriptors used in a model and the investigated endpoint. This task can be also solved using recently developed drug-like descriptors [36]. The concept of drug-like properties is a hot topic currently [36]. Drug-like descriptors brought to light the understanding of the behavior of chemicals in living organism in the terms of absorption, distribution, metabolism, and excretion (ADME) processes, which are related to pharmacokinetic and/or pharmacodynamics processes [37,38]. Therefore, in the current study, we applied the drug-like descriptors related to FDs and considered the correlation between these descriptors and binding activity. Moreover, the understanding of the relationship between the chemical descriptors (which express electronic, topological, geometrical, and other properties) and substituents (functional groups) of FDs was the focus of the current investigation.

In the article by Andrew Worth «The future of *in silico* chemical safety ... and beyond», it was pointed out that the new term that has gained acceptance is *in chemico*, referring to abiotic assays that measure chemical reactivity (toward proteins) [39]. Therefore, in the current article, the binding activity of studied FDs with functional groups was explored in terms of possible toxic and pharmacological impact. We suppose that investigation of the binding activity of FDs can bring a new knowledge to the global activity of this class of chemicals covering a possible activity with 1117 disease-related proteins. The present study paves a way to select the most significant interactions between FDs and proteins and then to perform an individual testing of the best FDs. The article was also focused on the main groups of proteins and their role in living organisms.

A comprehensive interpretation of a large dataset of 169 FDs requires an understanding about the content of the dataset related to a type of functional groups connected to fullerene core. In the current study, the FDs were classified depending on the type of bonding to fullerene core. Then the analysis was made on the most active and the least active FDs based on the presence of functional groups. The investigated activity was expressed as binding score that demonstrates the ability of FDs to interact with certain proteins. The performed study demonstrated how structural changes of FDs lead to changes in investigated property (i.e., binding activity). A wide variety of 169 FDs' structures by different types and classes gave valuable information about the properties of FDs related to their potential application as drugs, simultaneously with evaluation of their potential safety/toxicity. To visualize the drug-related properties and safety/toxicity predictions, the techniques based on CPANN algorithm and

Kohonen networks were applied. A heatmap of binding scores for 169 FDs with 1117 disease-related proteins represents valuable information on the individual selection of possible drugs, together with information about the possible side effects and toxic properties of considered individual FDs. It should be noted that not only functional groups were the focus of our study, but also the level of hydrogenation (saturation) of FDs and its influence on binding activity.

Moreover, in this study, analysis of structural descriptors (drug-like descriptors) and their connection with structure and binding activity of FDs was done. Application of cheminformatics tools enabled explanation of some features of FDs affecting the binding activity.

2. Materials and Methods

2.1. Dataset

A large set of 169 fullerene derivatives (FDs), represented in our previous work [40], was explored in the current study. The list of 169 FDs is represented in the supplementary material section, Table S1 (pages S2–S61). The classification of FDs dependent on the type of bond related to substituent group attached to the fullerene C60 core is represented in Tables S2–S8 (pages S62–S87). The investigated FDs include fullerenes C60, C70, and C80.

In a previous work [40], the binding activity for 169 FDs related to 1117 proteins, expressed as a binding score (Bscores), were calculated. The proteins were extracted from the RCSB Protein Data Bank [41]. A heat map of the binding scores activity of 169 FDs with 1117 proteins is represented in supplementary material section as an Excel file "Suppl_Heat map 169 FD × 1117 Proteins". In this file the Bscores of 1117 proteins data were screened against 169 FDs, forming the color coding heatmap, where red-orange color corresponds to the highest value of Bscores, yellow—the moderate values, and green—the lowest values of Bscores.

Let us consider the overall characteristics of these 1117 disease-related proteins. It is well known that proteins perform many different functions within organisms, such as (a) catalyzing metabolic reactions; (b) DNA replication; (c) responding to stimuli, providing structure to cells and organisms; and (d) transporting molecules from one location to another. The proteins investigated in this study belong to different classes according to their functions. The short description of groups of proteins related to different functions in organism, in a broad sense, is represented in Table 1.

Table 1. A short description of groups of proteins investigated in this study related to different functions in organism.

Function of Proteins	Class of Proteins
(a) catalyzing metabolic reactions (b) DNA replication	ENZYMES: OXIDOREDUCTASE; HYDROLASE; ISOMERASES; TRANSFERASE; LYASE; LIGASE GENE REGULATION; TRANSCRIPTION
(c) responding to stimuli, providing structure to cells and organisms	MEMBRANE RECEPTOR PROTEIN; HORMONE RECEPTOR PROTEIN; IMMUNE SYSTEM PROTEIN; SIGNALING PROTEINS; GROWTH FACTORS; ANTIMICROBIAL ANTITUMOR PROTEINS; CELL ADHESION; BIOTIN-BINDING PROTEIN
(d) transporting molecules from one location to another	TRANSPORT PROTEIN; LIPID TRANSFER PROTEIN

The detailed description of the individual groups of proteins, listed in Table 1, is provided in the supplementary material section (page S89).

2.2. Descriptors

Twenty five descriptors generated with use of DataWarrior software (developed by Actelion Pharmaceuticals Ltd. (Allschwil, Switzerland) [42]) were employed in the study: H-acceptors, H-donors, total surface area, relative PSA, polar surface area, drug-likeness, Mol_weight, cLogP, cLogS, electronegative atoms, stereo centers, rotatable bonds, rings closures, small rings, aromatic rings, aromatic atoms, sp3-atoms, symmetric atoms, amides, amines, aromatic nitrogen, basic nitrogen, acidic oxygens, non-H atoms, non-C/H atoms. These descriptors are used in drug design to describe drug-like properties of chemicals. Additionally, two descriptors employed by authors [40]—polarizability in cubic angstroms (*QPpolrz*) and topological diameter (TD) characterized the size of molecules—were used in the study.

2.3. The Counter Propagation Artificial Neural Network (CPANN) Algorithm and Self-Organizing Kohonen Maps

The detailed description of CPANN employed in the current study is represented in the supplementary material section (pages S90–S91). The architecture of CPANN is shown in Figure 2S (page S90) and reported in papers [43–45].

The CPANN is basically a two-layer neural network. It consists of a Kohonen layer (influenced by the input (descriptors)) and an output layer (influenced by the target (binding activity—Bscores)). CPANNs can be used as lookup tables. There is a one-to-one correspondence between the neurons in the Kohonen map and those in the output map. The self-organizing Kohonen Maps, as a data visualization technique [46], was applied for visualization of structurally similar molecules that tend to have similar activities. In this work, the focus was on the relationship between descriptors and FDs binding activity. Moreover, the clusters of FDs with similar functional groups and structure were examined in relation to the binding activity. The description of the code used in this study and its applications are reported by Grošelj et al. [47].

2.4. A Self-Organizing Kohonen Network

Kohonen networks learn to create maps of the input space in a self-organizing way. The best-known and most popular model of self-organizing networks is the topology-preserving map proposed by Teuvo Kohonen [46]. Self-organizing maps (SOMs) belong to a group of neural networks that use unsupervised learning [46]. Unsupervised learning supports the arrangement of objects (proteins in the present work) in the input layer map based on the similarity among input variables (expressed as binding scores activity). There is no golden standard and no straightforward external validity testing in this case. Each SOM consists of a predefined number of neurons, where each neuron has an associated weight vector. The number of elements in each vector is equal to the dimensionality of the input space. In our study, we used 5×5 matrices. The similar objects placed in the same or closest neurons. In the study, the Kohonen network was applied for organization of 1117 proteins in 2D map, and the number of proteins was reduced by elimination of the most similar objects.

3. Results

3.1. Reduction of the Number of Proteins by Using Kohonen Network

In this part of study the matrix containing the binding activity, expressed as a binding scores (Bscores), for 1117 proteins related to 169 FDs was composed. The neural network with dimension 5×5 was trained for 100 learning epochs. A Kohonen map of 5×5 with the distribution of 1117 proteins was obtained. The objects (protein numbers) were distributed by similarity determined by the binding activity. For example, similar objects are located close to each other in the Kohonen map. The Euclidean distances for each of the proteins placed in individual neurons were calculated. The Figures with Euclidean distance vs. ID of proteins were placed in the supplementary material section "Selection of the most significant proteins" (pages S92–S112). In each neuron, the proteins with the smallest and largest Euclidean distances were selected. This operation was done to reduce the number of proteins and get a global generalized view. This helped to find the main classes of proteins which differ by their behavior related to the considered FDs. The number of proteins were reduced from 1117 to 57. The Kohonen map with distribution of 57 proteins is represented in Figure 1.

	1	2	3	4	5
5	2AEB-HYDROLASE 1OW3-GENE REGULATION	1K3U-LYASE 1HKN-GROWTH FACTOR	1SRE-BIOTIN-BINDING PROTEIN 1MQ0-HYDROLASE	1CZ2-LIPID TRASFER PROTEIN 1FYN-TRANSFERASE 1XY1-HORMONE	1EFR-HYDROLASE 2LGS-LIGASE 1OF7-OXIDOREDUCTASE
4	2BE1-TRANSCRIPTION 1PGP-OXIDOREDUCTASE	1HVL- HYDROLASE 1ENT- HYDROLASE	1IDA- HYDROLASE 1NCO- ANTIBACTERIAL AND ANTITUMOR PROTEIN	1CPS- HYDROLASE 2NCM - CELL ADHESION	1DB4-HYDROLASE 1H92-TRANSFERASE
3	1EEY- IMMUNE SYSTEM 1W6K-ISOMERASE 1OOQ-OXIDOREDUCTASE 1YAA-AMINOTRANSFERASE	1SFF-TRANSFERASE	1YPP-HYDROLASE 1DS6-SIGNALING PROTEIN	1AAQ-HYDROLASE 1HEF- HYDROLASE	1DB1-GENE REGULATION 1OYA-OXIDOREDUCTASE 1RML-GROWTH FACTOR 2BFW-TRANSFERASE
2	1JBQ-LYASE 2C6Q-OXIDOREDUCTASE 1RTD-TRANSFERASE/DNA	1J59-GENE REGULATION 1P93-HORMONE RECEPTOR 1CVI- HYDROLASE	2CKG-HYDROLASE 2PAW-TRANSFERASE 2BH9-OXIDOREDUCTASE	1TC1-TRANSFERASE 1DHF-OXIDOREDUCTASE	1S50-MEMBRANE PROTEIN 1YVJ-TRANSFERASE
1	1M9M-OXIDOREDUCTASE 1XFH- TRANSPORT PROTEIN	1R0W-TRANSPORT PROTEIN 1ILH-GENE REGULATION 1FO4-OXIDOREDUCTASE	2BCE-HYDROLASE	1JVM-MEMBRANE PROTEIN	1SM2-TRANSFERASE 2EU9-TRANSFERASE
	1	2	3	4	5

Figure 1. The Kohonen map (5 × 5) with distribution of 57 proteins.

The substances like FDs can interact with proteins in a different way, depending on the type of proteins and their function, and can cause the appropriate changes in system. The interaction of proteins with FDs can lead to (a) change in catalyzing the metabolic reactions in organism; (b) chemical changes to the genetic material; (c) change in responding to stimuli, providing structure to cells and organisms; or (d) change in transporting molecules from one location to another.

The obtained Kohonen map in Figure 1 contains enzymes (red color), receptors (violet color), gene regulation or transcription (green color), and transport proteins (blue color).

3.2. Selection of Characteristic for Binding Activity

The comprehensive multi-software protein-ligand docking simulation and chemoinformatics approaches were applied to investigate the interaction of 1117 proteins with 169 FD nanoparticles, which was reported first in the work [40]. The binding score (Bscores) parameter is responsible for several types of intermolecular interactions and apprises the force of interaction between protein and ligand (FD). Firstly, the average value of Bscores for 1117 proteins (marked as Average sum) calculated for each of 169 FDs was found. Secondly, a top 110 proteins that possessed the highest binding activity was selected and determined the average Bscores for these 110 proteins (marked as Average110). Thirdly, the average Bscores for 57 proteins was determined through selection from the Kohonen map (marked as Average 57). These 57 proteins cover the main functions in the existing dataset (see Figure 1).

The structures of FDs were expressed as two descriptors: Polarizability in cubic angstroms ($QPpolrz$) and topological diameter (TD) selected in our previous study [40].

Then, the correlation between Average sum (for 1117 proteins), Average 110, Average 57, and $QPpolrz$ and TD was the focus of the investigation. The results are shown in Table 2.

Table 2. The correlation between Average sum, Average 110, Average 57, polarizability (QPpolrz), and topological diameter (TD)

Av_Bscores/Descriptors	Average Sum	Average 110	Average 57	QPpolrz	TD
Average sum	1	0.995	0.977	0.947	0.899
Average110	0.995	1	0.974	0.964	0.885
Average57	0.977	0.974	1	0.908	0.889
QPpolrz	0.947	0.964	0.908	1	0.837
TD	0.899	0.885	0.889	0.837	1

Obtained results demonstrated that average Bscores for the 1117 proteins, the top 110 proteins, and for 57 proteins are highly correlated with the structure of FDs expressed as two descriptors: QPpolrz and TD.

In the next step, the Average sum for all 1117 proteins was used as a characterization of binding activity of FDs and marked as "Av Bscores".

3.3. The Characteristics of FDs Dataset with Relation to Binding Activity

The current list of FDs covers many classes of chemical compounds. In this section the binding activity was expressed as average binding scores (Av Bscores) and considered here in the range from 4000 to 8000. The distribution of 169 FDs dependent on their binding activity (Av Bscores) is represented in Figure 2.

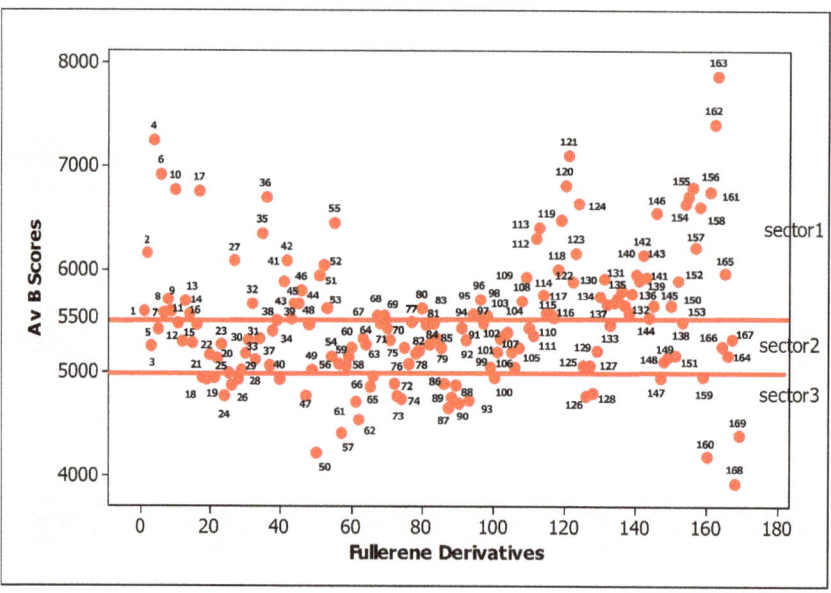

Figure 2. The distribution of fullerene derivatives according to their binding activities.

The FDs with binding scores in the range 5500 to 8000 are the most active (sector 1). The interval 5500 to 5000 belongs to the moderately active FDs (sector 2). The majority of FDs are located in this sector. The least active or low active FDs have the binding activity in the scale of 5000 to 4000 (sector 3).

The goal of this work was to illustrate how functional groups of FDs influence on the binding activity (Av Bscore) of FDs. The FDs were considered in the order of decreasing the Bscores values.

The classification of FDs depending on the type of bond of substituent groups attached to the fullerene C60 core with indication of the level of binding activity is represented in the supplementary material (SI) section, Tables S2–S8 (pages S62–S87). The considered dataset of FDs contains the FDs substituent groups attached to C60 core with (1) single bond containing alkyl groups; (2) cyclopropane three-membered ring; (3) pyrrolidine (five-membered ring) or pyridine (six-membered) heterocycles containing nitrogen; (4) six-membered (cyclohexane) ring; (5) benzene (aromatic six-membered) ring; (6) fused pair of six-membered rings; and (7) bridged bicycle rings which are illustrated in Tables S2–S8.

3.4. The Characteristics of the Least Active and the Most Active FDs

The lowest value of binding activity belongs to pristine fullerene C60. The surface of C60 fullerene contains 20 hexagons and 12 pentagons, where all rings are fused, all double bonds are conjugated. In spite of their extreme conjugation, they behave chemically and physically as electron-deficient alkenes rather than electron rich aromatic systems [48]. The least active FDs are shown in Table 3.

Table 3. The summary table for the least active fullerenes and fullerene derivatives without functional groups or with a minimal number of them.

FD_ID	3D Structure	Mol. Formula and/or Functional Groups	Binding Score Bscores	Difference in Bscores from C60
FD168		C_{60}	3938.3	0
FD50		C_{70}	4224.3	286
FD169		$C_{80}H_2$	4398.5	461
FD160		$C_{60}H_4O_4$ $C_{60}(OH)_4$ 4 hydroxyl groups –OH	4192.2	254
FD57		$C_{62}H_2O_2$ C_{60}-CH-COOH	4412.7	475
FD61		$C_{60}H_{54}O_{20}$ $C_{60}H_{34}(OH)_{20}$ 20 hydroxyl groups –OH	4725.1	787
FD93		$C_{60}H_{50}O_{24}$ $C_{60}H_{26}(OH)_{24}$ 24 hydroxyl groups –OH	4735.3	797

The FDs without functional groups or with only few hydroxyl –OH groups or carboxyl groups –COOH demonstrated the lowest binding activity (Bscores), approximately less than 5000.

Table 3 also shows the differences between the binding activity (Bscore) of pristine fullerene C_{60} and the least active fullerenes.

The least active is fullerene C_{60} (**FD168** = 3938.3). The differences in binding activity between C_{60} (**FD68** = 3938.3) and C_{70} (**FD50** = 4224.3) was equal to 286, and between C_{60} (**FD168** = 3938.3) and $C_{80}H_2$ (**FD169** = 4398.5) was equal to 460.2. The addition of four hydroxyl groups (–OH) in **FD160** (4192.2) resulted the increase of binding activity by 253.9 in comparison with C_{60} (**FD168** = 3938.3). The binding activity of saturated **FD61** (4725.1) containing 20 hydroxyl groups is greater by 786.8 in comparison with C_{60} (**FD168** = 3938.3). Approximately the same rise of binding activity, equal to 797, in comparison with C_{60} (**FD168** = 3938.3) was obtained for **FD93** (4735.3) containing 24 hydroxyl groups. The activity of **FD93** (4735.3) containing 24 –OH, in comparison with **FD61** (4725.1) containing 20 –OH, was increased only by 10. We can suggest that in this case the presence of –OH has influence on activity, but the level of saturation of considered FDs should be taken into consideration too. Thus, the higher level of saturation of **FD61** (C60H34(OH)20) containing 34 hydrogens in C60 core) in comparison with **FD93** (C60H26(OH)24), containing 26 hydrogens in C60 core) can cause the reduction of binding activity of **FD93**. Increasing the binding activity of **FD93** caused by the additional four hydroxyl groups –OH can be overlapped with decreasing activity due to a lower level of saturation (26-H in **FD93** in comparison with 34-H in **FD61**).

Allen and co-workers conducted investigations in order to determine the antioxidant activity of a range of fullerenes (i.e., C60, C70, and fullerene soot) and then ranked them according to their comparative efficiency. They proposed the following sequence of antioxidant efficiency: C70 > C 60/C70 (80/20) > C60/C70 (93/7) > C60 [49]. The binding activity of C70 in comparison with C60 was higher by 286. In addition, we supposed that theoretically calculated Bscores can also be an indicator of antioxidant activity of FDs.

The differences in binding activity (ΔBscores) between the most active FDs and pristine fullerene C_{60} are represented in the . The presence of the most active groups in FDs lead to an increase of binding activity in comparison with pristine fullerene C_{60} by 2162–3947. Thus, the differences in binding activity (ΔBscores) of the moderate to least active FDs in comparison with pristine fullerene C_{60}, approximately, is in the range 2162–475.

Analyzing data represented in the supplementary material (SI) section in Tables S2–S8 (pages S62–S87), one can notice that the most active **FD6** has the longest alkyl chain with the alkenyl group (double unsaturated C = C-) in the middle of the chain (see Group 1 (page S62)). Group 2 (pages S64–S65), containing two benzene rings, had high activity. In Group 2c (page S67) the activity was caused by presence of ammonium groups (**FDs 163, 162, 161**), and in Group 2d (page S67) by presence of phosphonate groups **FDs 158, 165**. Aromatic nitrogen in Group 3a (pages S70–S71) caused the high activity for **FDs 154–157** and **112, 113**. Pyridine rings as well as benzene rings, probably, contribute to the high binding activity in Group 3c (pages S73–S74) (see **FDs 35** and **36**).

FDs 118–124 in group 5b (page S80) possessed high activity due to presence of 8–14 NO_2 groups. FDs from the Group 5e (page S85) experienced high activity due to presence of pyridine groups (**FDs 35, 36**).

The analysis of the activity of clusters of considered FDs is given below using visualization tools in 2D Kohonen maps, which is complemented with analysis of structural drug-like descriptors correlated with the binding activity.

3.5. CPANN Model Based on Drug-Like Descriptors

3.5.1. Selection of Drug-Like Properties Descriptors for Modelling

Drug-likeness is a qualitative concept used in drug design related to bioavailability of substances. It is estimated from the molecular structure. Drug-likeness may be defined as a complex balance of various molecular properties and structure features which determine whether a particular molecule is similar to the known drugs. We notice the absence of studies about drug-likeness of FDs. DataWarrior software developed by Actelion Pharmaceuticals Ltd. [43] has been used to calculate drug-like descriptors for FDs. Analysis of drug-like properties of FDs can be related to the novelty of our study.

Between properties considered for drug-likeness, we can highlight that the hydrophobicity, electronic distribution, hydrogen bonding characteristics, molecule size and flexibility, and of course, the presence of various pharmacophore features influence the behavior of molecule in a living organism, including bioavailability, transport properties, affinity to proteins, reactivity, toxicity, metabolic stability, and many others. The concept of drug-likeness provides useful guidelines for early-stage drug discovery [37,50]. It contains the analysis of the observed distribution of some key physicochemical properties of approved drugs, including molecular weight, hydrophobicity, and polarity related to known drugs [38]. These parameters are well known and applicable in drug design. This is why it is sensible to use these criteria in the study of a new class of chemicals, like FDs, to find some features understandable for drug design researchers and for future examination of a unique class of chemicals that are promising for application in drug design. The assessment of drug-likeness is known as Lipinski's rule of five (Ro5), where simple count criteria (like limits for molecular weight, log P, or number of hydrogen bond donors or acceptors) and others were used [51].

Twenty-five drug-like descriptors were calculated using DataWarrior software [42]. These descriptors are reported in the section "Materials and Methods". The "drug-like" properties include the structural features and physicochemical properties. These properties can be used for characterization of pharmacophore: A substituent in FDs or a part of a molecular structure that is responsible for particular biological or pharmacological interaction [52].

3.5.2. CP ANN Model Based on 27 Descriptors

The CPANN model developed in this section was based on twenty-seven molecular descriptors. First, twenty-five descriptors were generated by DataWarrior software, where all calculated descriptors are drug-like properties of compounds. These descriptors can be used to explore some properties that might play a role in formation of the interaction between the ligand (FD) and receptor (protein). Two descriptors *QPpolrz* and *TD* that were applied in the previous study [40] were added in the current study.

The CPANN models based on the generated drug-like descriptors were trained. The input data for 169 FDs were normalized. The optimal model was obtained with dimension 20 × 20 and number of learning epochs equal to 100. The model demonstrated the following statistical performance for the whole data set that was used as a training set: squared regression coefficient, $R^2 = 0.96$, (RMSE = 0.21), leave-one-out cross-validation (LOO-CV) regression coefficient, $Q^2_{cv} = 0.87$, (RMSE = 0.22). The internal validation of CPANN models was performed using the LOO-CV procedure for evaluation of the quality and goodness of fit of the model [53,54].

It should be highlighted that the developed model was used for visualization of the whole dataset of FDs and to study the correlation and relationships between descriptors and binding activity.

3.5.3. Analysis of Distribution of FDs in the Top Map of the CPANN Model Based on 27 Descriptors

The distribution of FDs in the top map 20 × 20 of the CPANN model based on 27 descriptors overlapped with the output layer, with distribution of values of binding activity, is represented in Figure 3.

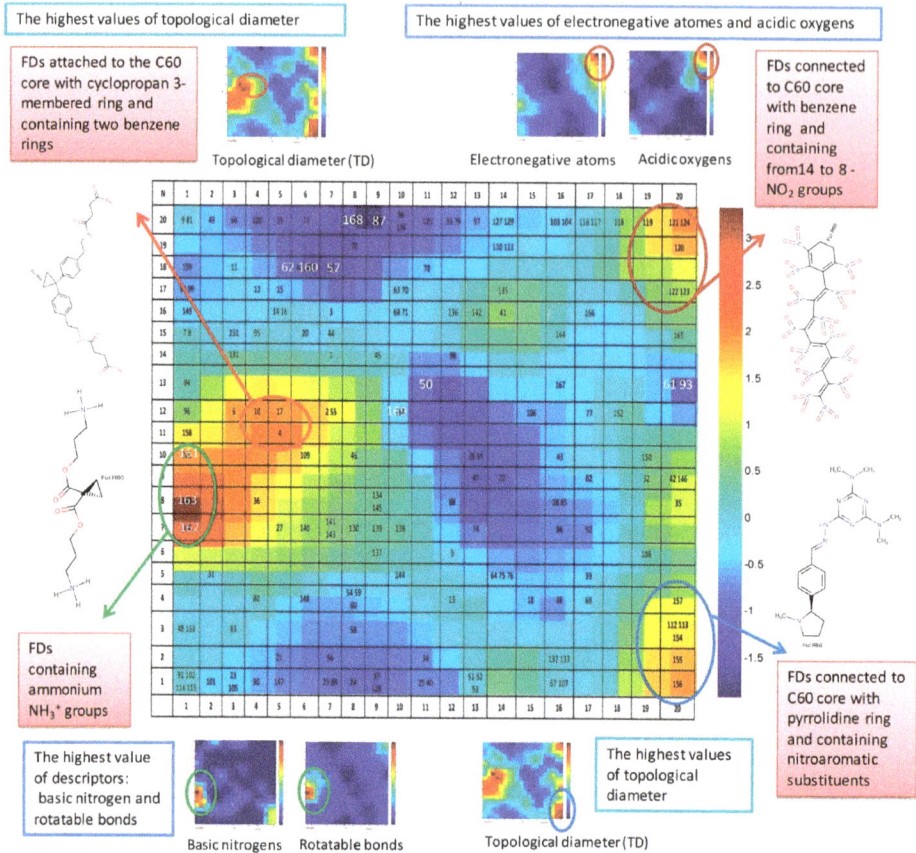

Figure 3. The distribution of FDs in the top map 20 × 20 of the CPANN model based on 27 descriptors overlapped with the output layer with binding activity.

The blue color in Figure 3 corresponds to the lowest value of binding activity (Bscores) and the red color to the highest values. The scale bar represents the normalized data of Bscores. The top map in Figure 3 is complemented with illustration of some of the most active groups of FDs and weight maps of related descriptors that have extreme values for these selected groups of FDs. The most active group of FDs located in neurons 1 × (7,8,10) contain ammonium NH_3^+ groups. This area corresponds to the highest value of descriptors: basic nitrogen and rotatable bonds. See the weight maps of basic nitrogen and rotatable bonds at the left bottom corner in Figure 3.

The active group of FDs attached to the C60 core with cyclopropane three-membered ring and containing two benzene rings is located in neurons 4 × 12 and 5 × (11,12). This group of FDs corresponds to the area with the highest values of topological diameter descriptor. The weight map of the topological diameter descriptor is shown at the left top corner in Figure 3.

The group of FDs connected to C60 core with benzene ring and containing from 14 to 8 NO_2 groups belongs to the most active FDs too, and is located in the right top corner of top map in neurons 20 × (20,19,17) and 19 × 19. These groups of FDs are characterized by the highest values of descriptors: electronegative atoms and acidic oxygen. The weight maps of pointed descriptors are shown at the right top side in Figure 3.

The next active group of FDs contains the FDs connected to C60 core with pyrrolidine ring and containing nitro aromatic substituents. This group of FDs is shown in Figure 3 at the right bottom corner of the top map. The highest values of the topological diameter descriptor correspond to this area, which was highlighted in the weigh map located close to this group from the right bottom side of Figure 3.

Of course, Figure 3 only partly demonstrates the characterization of some groups of FDs and the related descriptors that play the most significant role only for these groups.

To clarify this statement, let us consider the most active FDs with the highest value of Bscores. These are **FD162** and **FD163**, containing 6 and 8 ammonium NH_3^+ groups, correspondingly, and located in neurons 1 × (7,8). These FDs possess the highest value of molecular weight, rotatable bonds, sp3 atoms, amines, basic nitrogen, non-H atoms, and polarizability QPpolrz.

The lowest value of binding activity (Bscores) corresponds to pristine fullerene **FD168** (C60) located on neuron 8 × 20. The fullerene C60 possesses the lowest total surface area, molecular weight, rotatable bonds, electronegative atoms, sp3 atoms, polarizability QPpolrz, and topological diameter. Thus, C60 does not have functional groups or substituents and can be used a reference molecule for comparison with other FDs containing functional groups related to binding activity.

The present section demonstrated only a quick simplified look on information about the relationship between FDs, their property (BScores), and applied descriptors supported by visualization tools (particularly CPANN).

3.5.4. Consensus Model Based on 10 Descriptors

The key task of QSAR models is the selection of a minimal set of descriptors correlated with the studied property of an organic compound [55]. Reduction of the number of descriptors was performed using the Kohonen mapping technique. This method is based on selection of descriptors from the same neuron with the greatest and smallest Euclidian distances, as the inherent property of the Kohonen map is the position of the same or similar objects at the same or closest neurons.

Selection of descriptors was made using a 2 × 2 Kohonen map. Eight (8) descriptors were selected: cLogS, sp3-atoms, drug-likeness, aromatic atoms, electronegative atoms, rotatable bonds, amides, basic nitrogen.

The consensus model was built using eight drug-like properties descriptors plus two descriptors from previous study of polarizability in cubic angstroms and topological diameter (QPpolrz and TD) [40]. The input data were normalized. Binding activity (Bscores) were used as a response. The optimal selected model with architecture 20 × 20 was trained for 100 learning epochs.

The model demonstrated a high level of accuracy with R^2 = 0.95 and leave-one-out test cross-validation 0.92.

The output layers for responses were used in the study as weight maps, for demonstration of distribution of these parameters in 2D space, for comparison with distribution of applied descriptors. This technique represents the distribution of multidimensional parameters in 2D space and allows for analysis of the similarities or correlation between studied parameters.

The consensus CPANN model mentioned above was used for visualization of molecular space in 2D maps, and analysis of the distribution of FD molecules decorated with different functional groups related to different binding activity. The top map 20 × 20 of the CPANN model based on 10 descriptors with distribution of FDs overlapped with the output layer of binding activity (Bscores) is represented in Figure 4.

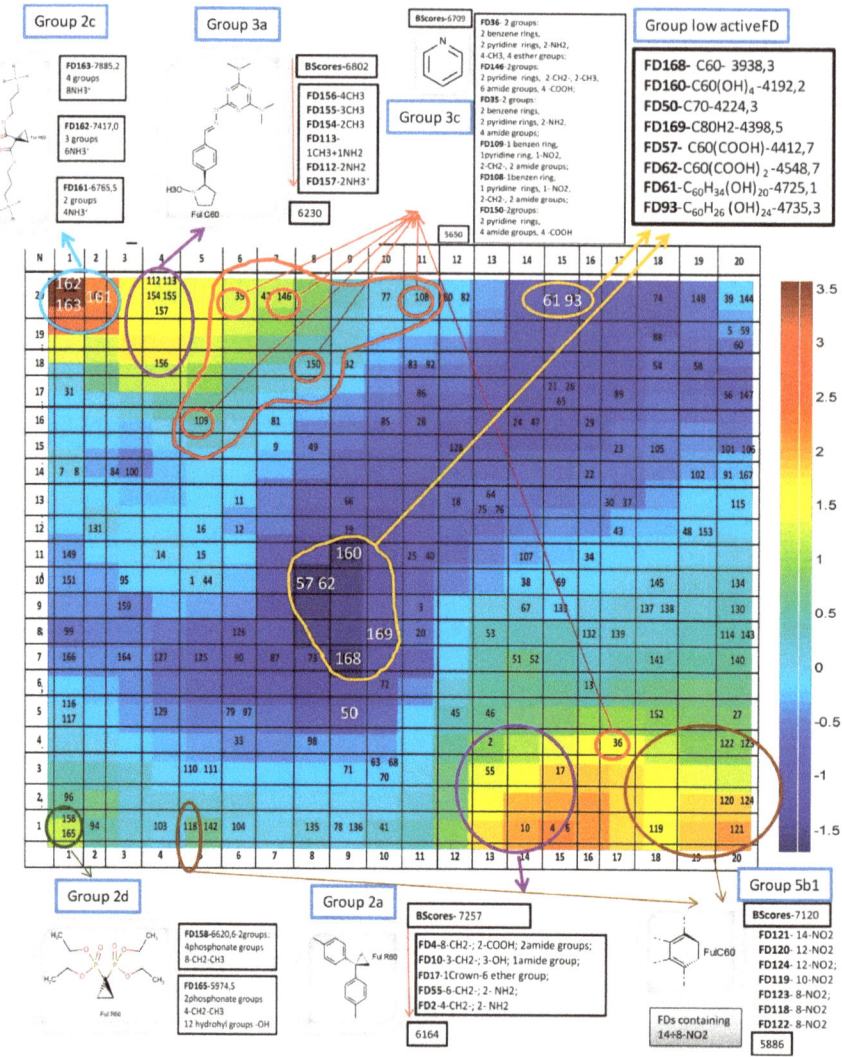

Figure 4. The top map 20 × 20 of the consensus model based on 10 descriptors with distribution of FDs overlapped with the output layer of binding activity (Bscores), with indication of the most active groups of FDs as well as the FDs with lowest activity.

3.5.5. Analysis of Distribution of FDs in the Top Map of the Consensus Model Based on 10 Descriptors.

The top map was complemented with illustration of some of the most active groups of FDs as well as the FDs with lowest activity.

The color in the map (Figure 4) depends on the binding activity. The red one was related to the most active space (the highest value of BScores), while the dark blue area corresponded to the least active FDs, having the lowest value of Bscores.

The classification of FDs dependent on type of bond of substituent groups attached to the fullerene C60 core with detailed characterization of activity (A-active, M-moderate active, and L-low active) is represented in the supplementary information (SI) section, in Tables S2–S8 (pages S62–S87).

The most active groups of FDs shown in the Figure 4 are described below. Group 2 is located in Table S3 (page S64). For reference see group 2a (Group 2a attached to the C60 core with cyclopropane three-membered ring and containing two benzene rings with level of activity 7257–6164) (pages S64–65); group 2c (Group 2c attached to the C60 core with cyclopropane three-membered ring and containing ammonium groups with level of activity 7885–6766), and 2d (Group 2d attached to the C60 core with cyclopropane three-membered ring and containing phosphonate groups with level of activity 6621–5975) (page S67).

Group 3 is located in Table S4 (page S70). For reference see group 3a (Group 3a attached to the C60 core with pyrrolidine (five-membered ring) and containing aromatic nitrogen with level of activity 6802–6230) (pages S70–71); group 3c (Group 3c attached to the C60 core with six-membered cycle and containing in the side chain pyridine ring or attached to the C60 core with pyridine ring or six-membered heterocycle containing nitrogen with level of activity 6709–5650) (page S73–74).

Group 5 is located in Table S6 (page S78). Group 5b1 (Group 5b1—the most active FDs connected to C60 core with benzene ring and containing 8–14 nitro groups -NO2 with activity 7120–5886) (page S80).

The low active FDs are located in the center of the Kohonen map (Blue area) and are listed in the top right corner, with indication of the level of their activity expressed as Bscores.

3.6. The Characterization of Drug-Like Descriptors Related to Binding Activity

3.6.1. Results of Principle Component Analysis for 25 Drug-Like descriptors

The principle component analysis (PCA) was performed for 25 drug-like descriptors. The role of descriptors is illustrated at the loading plot for the first two components where the loadings for the second component (y-axis) are plotted versus the loadings for the first component (x-axis). A line is drawn from each loading to the (0, 0) point. The loading plot represented in Figure 5 represents a good visualization for 25 drug-like descriptors and their relation to each other. The highly correlated descriptors with CC from 1 to 0.895 are located on the right side of the plot, labeled as red lines. The aromatic atoms and aromatic rings, which have the negative correlation with sp3-atoms and stereo centers are located in opposite side from 0.0 in Figure 5. The cLogP is located opposite to total surface area.

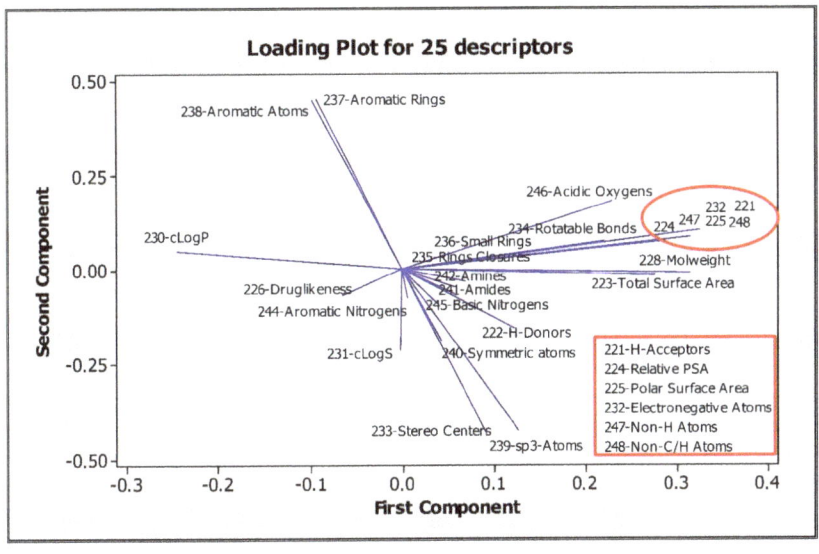

Figure 5. The loading plot for 25 drug-like descriptors.

In the study below the correlation between these descriptors was performed using weight maps of CPANN models and by calculating correlation coefficient using the Minitab program.

3.6.2. How Drug-Like Descriptors Correlated to Binding Activity

The correlation between some of drug-like descriptors is represented in Figure 6. First of all, the Pearson correlation coefficients (CC) were calculated for all applied descriptors as well as for binding activity (Bscores) using Minitab software. The correlation coefficients (CC) between considered descriptors greater than 0.6 are listed in the supplementary material (SI) section, in Table S9 (page S113).

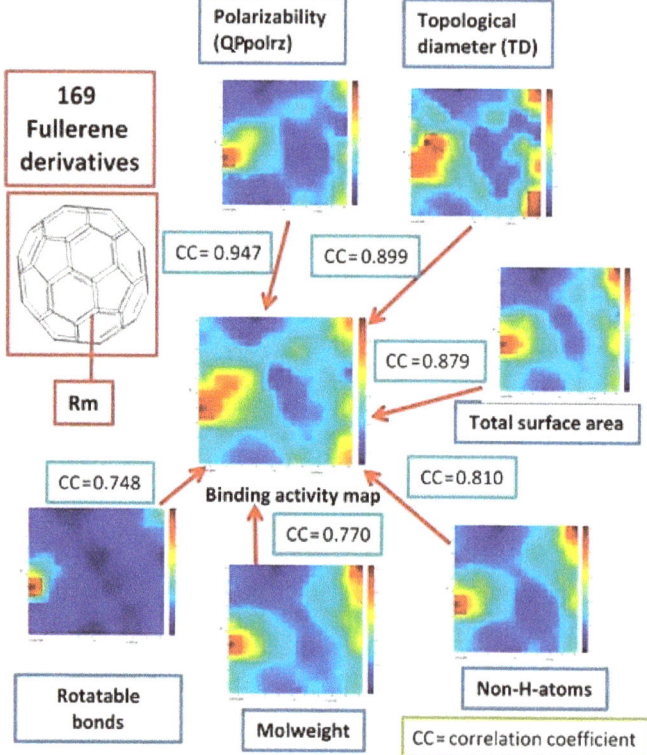

Figure 6. The correlation between drug-like descriptors and binding activity. Weight maps and correlation coefficients (CC).

The study demonstrated that the binding activity (Bscores) is highly correlated with polarizability (CC = 0.947) and topological diameter (CC = 0.899). Then, by the level of correlation, follow the total surface area (CC = 0.879), non-H-atoms (CC = 0.810), mol. weight (CC = 0.770) and rotatable bonds (0.748).

The polarizability (*QPpolrz*), topological diameter (*TD*), total surface area, non H-atoms, mol. weight can be used for characterization of pharmacokinetic events, which are connected with such phenomenon as permeation, which depends mainly on size and shape, and on lipophilicity or hydrophobicity, which encodes recognition forces such as hydrophobic interactions, H-bonding capacity, and van der Waals forces (i.e., polarity). They also connected with recognition by proteins that have evolved to be promiscuous (i.e., to bind structurally quite diverse xenobiotics), for example, drug-metabolizing enzymes, xenobiotic transporters, and serum proteins. Here the molecular properties, such as hydrophobicity and H-bonding capacity, play a major role, together with some fuzzy pharmacophores defined by the presence of a small number of recognition groups.

The descriptor number of rotatable bonds belongs to characteristics of pharmacodynamic events that result from interaction with biological targets, such as receptors, endobiotic-metabolizing enzymes, ion channels, nucleic acids, and so on. Such events are initiated when bioactive agents are recognized by (i.e., bind to) their respective target, a recognition that depends mainly, if not exclusively, on a pharmacophore site within the protein target. In other words, pharmacodynamics events are highly dependent on 3D structure.

Moreover, the descriptor number of rotatable bonds contains the information about compound's conformational space. This implicit information is remarkable in suggesting that conformational behavior matters, not only in pharmacodynamics events (drug target recognition), but also from an ADME perspective [52].

3.6.3. The Descriptors Related to Aromaticity

The aromaticity plays a crucial role in drug design. The authors in [56] investigated the impact of aromatic ring count (the number of aromatic and heteroaromatic rings) in molecules against various developability parameters—aqueous solubility, lipophilicity, serum albumin binding, CyP450 inhibition, and human Ether-à-go-go-Related Gene (hERG) inhibition. It was also demonstrated that even within a defined lipophilicity range, increased aromatic ring count leads to decreased aqueous solubility [56].

In the present study, the special focus was made on correlation of aromatic rings and atoms related to FDs. Lipophilicity was expressed as LogP in our study. A weak correlation for aromatic atoms and aromatic rings with LogP (CC = 0.249–0.268) was obtained. The solubility was expressed as LogS and the inverse correlation was obtained for aromatic atoms and aromatic rings with LogS (CC = −0.466/−0.448), which also demonstrated that, in the case of FDs, an increased aromatic ring count leads to decreased aqueous solubility.

Figure 7 represents weight maps for correlated descriptors: aromatic atoms, aromatic rings, sp3-atoms, and stereo centers.

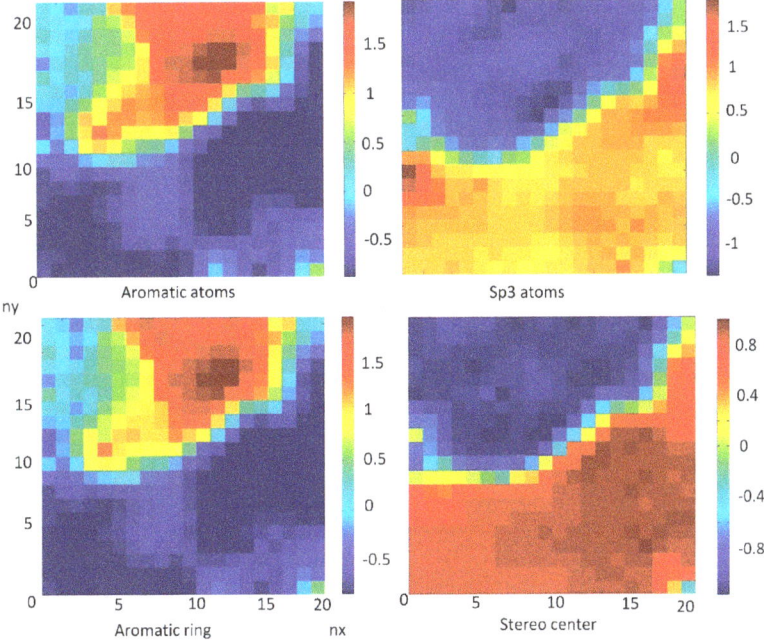

Figure 7. Weight maps for correlated descriptors for aromatic rings and atoms: aromatic atoms, aromatic rings, sp3-atoms, and stereo centers.

The aromatic atoms correlated with aromatic rings (CC = 0.996). The characterization of the aromatic nature of chemicals here was connected with two main descriptors: sp3-atoms and stereo centers, which are strongly correlated (CC = 0.979). It should be noted that aromatic atoms and aromatic rings have an inverse strong correlation with sp3-atoms and stereo centers (CC = −0.847/−0.852).

Descriptors: sp3-atoms and stereo centers were used to describe the saturation level of FDs, which are separately discussed in the article below.

3.6.4. The Role of LogP on Properties of FDs Inversely Correlated with Polar Surface Area

The weight maps of cLogP, which is inversely correlated with relative PSA (CC = −0.861) and polar surface area (CC = −0.797), are shown in the Figure 8.

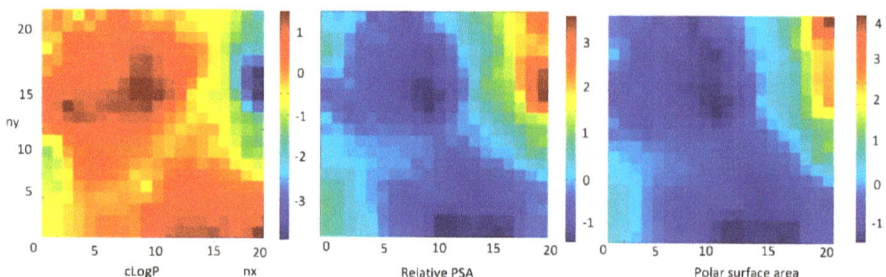

Figure 8. Weight maps of inversely correlated cLogP with polar surface area (PSA) and relative PSA.

The most commonly used measure of lipophilicity is the LogP parameter. This is, the partition coefficient of a molecule between aqueous and lipophilic phases, usually octanol and water. Lipophilicity is one of the most important physicochemical properties of a drug. It plays a role in solubility, absorption, membrane penetration, plasma protein binding, distribution, CNS penetration and partitioning into other tissues or organs, such as the liver, and has an impact on the routes of clearance. It is important in ligand recognition, not only to the target protein, but also in CYP450 interactions, hERG binding, and PXR-mediated enzyme induction.

The LogP value of a compound, which is the logarithm of its partition coefficient between n-octanol and water log ($c_{octanol}/c_{water}$), is a well-established measure of the compound's hydrophilicity. Low hydrophilicities and; therefore, high LogP values cause a poor absorption or permeation. Both descriptors characterize the *pharmacokinetic* events in a living organism.

It can be concluded that the FDs with a high relative PSA have a low value of LogP. This feature is important in the process of the selection chemicals suitable for drugs.

The authors in [57] reported that increased LogP improves the permeability of chemicals. However, increasing the LogP decreases the solubility and increase the toxicity.

3.7. *Investigation of Level of Hydrogenation (Saturation) of FDs*

Next, the dataset of 169 FDs used in the study was separated into 75 unsaturated FDs and 94 saturated FDs. According to the IUPAC nomenclature [58,59], the fully saturated fullerenes, like $C_{60}H_{60}$, belong to fullerenes.

Figure 9 demonstrated that saturated FDs can be separated from unsaturated FDs using the stereo center and sp3-atoms descriptors.

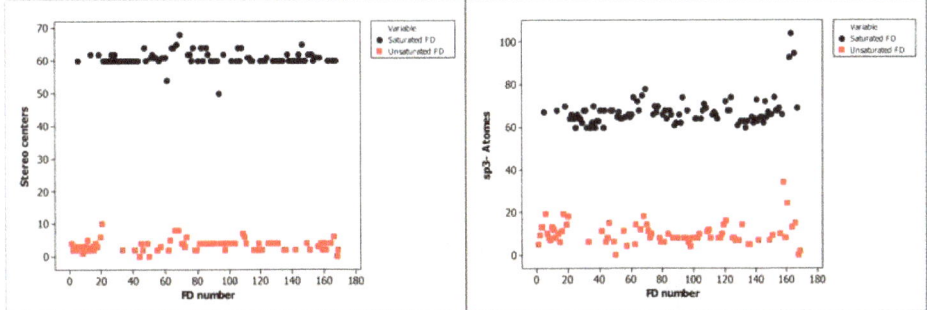

Figure 9. The distribution of saturated and unsaturated FDs depending on the stereo center and sp3-atoms descriptors.

These two descriptors are crucial in drug design. According to Lovering et al. [60], the Fsp3 (carbon bond saturation) is defined as the number of sp3 hybridized carbons/total carbon count. This descriptor correlates with melting point and solubility. The presence of stereo centers as well as a number of chiral centers are descriptors of complexity [60]. Saturation or hydrogenation depends on the amount of hydrogen atoms in FDs, and there is not clear separation on saturated and unsaturated. Only the lower limits are well determined. For saturated FDs, the limit corresponds to sp3 greater than 60. For unsaturated FDs, it corresponds to sp3 = 0.

Thus, the lowest sp3 value = 0 which corresponds to **FD168** (C60) and **FD50** (C70) with zero sp3 atoms. It should be noted that the pristine fullerene C60 is composed of sp^2 hybridized carbon nanostructures. Since the discovery of C60 by Kroto et al., the zero-dimensional carbon nanostructure has attracted increasing attention from scientists due to its unique structure and physical properties. A fullerene can act as an electron acceptor because the fullerene molecule requires that the C–C bonds interact through bent sp^2 hybridized carbon atoms, which leads to a strained structure with good reactivity. The curved π-conjugation of C60 within the unique sp^2 hybridized carbon atoms shows both π-character and substantial s-character, which is remarkably different from the planar π-conjugation within graphite and planar polycyclic aromatic hydrocarbons that are solely of π-character [61]. Due to the unsaturated character of the C–C bonds in the fullerene, there are plenty of electronic states to accept electrons from appropriate donors forming donor–π–acceptor combinations [62]. In drug design, two simple and interpretable measures of the complexity of molecules, prepared as potential drug candidates, were proposed. The first is carbon bond saturation, as defined by fraction sp3 (Fsp3), where Fsp3 = (number of sp3 hybridized carbons/total carbon count). The second is simply whether a chiral carbon exists in the molecule. It was demonstrated that both complexity (as measured by Fsp3) and the presence of chiral centers correlate with success as compounds transition from discovery, through clinical testing, to drugs. Moreover, it was shown that saturation correlates with solubility, an experimental physical property important to success in the drug discovery setting.

In the study of [63] it was assumed that compounds with higher solubility, higher permeability, and lower protein binding receive higher developability scores, whereas compounds with lower solubility, lower solubility, and higher protein binding receive lower developability scores. Low developability compounds, in turn, are associated with higher values of the aromatic descriptors and lower values of Fsp3. These descriptors are especially important for the large and lipophilic molecules (MW > 400, cLogP > 4).

It should be pointed out that FDs molecular weight (MW) is in the range of large molecules (MW = 720–1659). We supposed that FDs should be considered in drug design separately, according to unique properties and structure [64]. The special focus should be directed to sp2 hybridization of carbon in the molecule of fullerene C60.

It was demonstrated above that there is a strong correlation between sp3-atoms and stereo centers (CC = 0.979). Figure 10 demonstrated the inverse correlation between aromatic atoms and sp3-atoms (CC = −0.852), while number of saturated FDs was correlated with sp3-atoms (CC = 0,978) and inversely correlated with aromatic atoms (CC = −0.846).

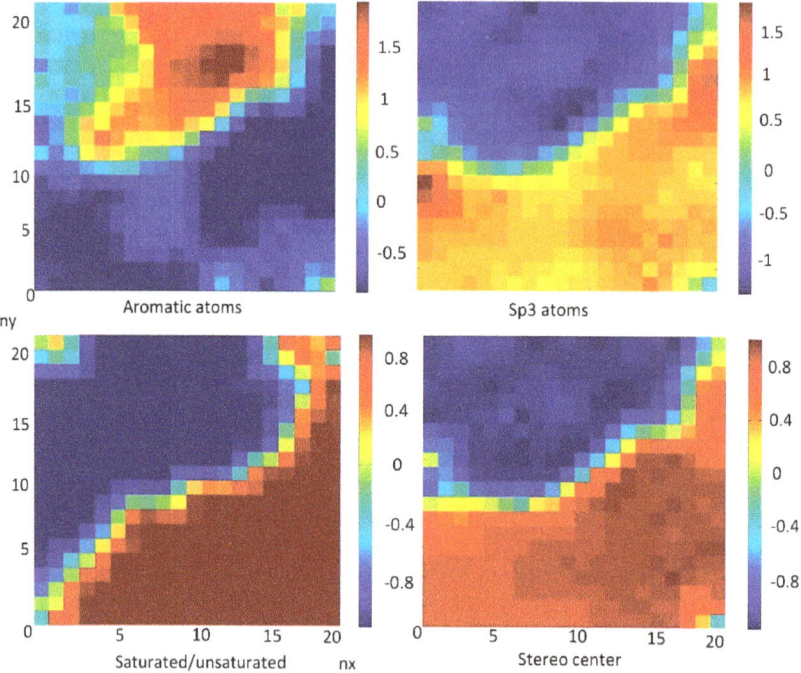

Figure 10. Weight maps of descriptors: aromatic atoms, sp3 atoms, stereo centers with distribution of saturated/unsaturated FDs.

In drug design [40,56,65] it is more desirable to shift the balance toward less aromatic and more aliphatic characteristics [56]. It is promisingly to study FDs because their structure contains sp2 carbons. The descriptors of sp3 atoms and inversely correlated aromatic atoms can help in the search for the most promising compounds suitable in drug design.

The question was aroused about the differences in the binding activity of saturated vs. unsaturated FDs. The saturated and unsaturated FDs having the same substituent (functional group) were selected from our dataset, and were placed in the supplementary material (SI) section, Table S10 (pages S114–S116). Table S10 contains the structural formula of considered FD molecules and functional groups, molecular formula, values of descriptors: QPpolrz, TD and Av_BScores.

In most cases the saturated fullerenes with the same functional groups had a larger binding affinity than the unsaturated fullerenes. The considered FDs had differences between saturated and non-saturated ones in the range of Bscore 93.99–175.79.

4. Conclusions

The goal of the current study was to characterize the binding activity related to 169 FDs using various cheminformatics tools. It was assumed that the global tendency in binding activity and the application of the special molecular descriptors used in drug design related to topological, electrical, and others properties of studied molecules can contribute to pharmacology or toxicology.

In this study, a classification of FDs was created based on bonding of substituent groups to the C60 core. The following substituent groups were considered:

1. Single bond containing alkyl groups;
2. Cyclopropane three-membered ring;
3. Pyrrolidine (five-membered ring) or pyridine (six-membered) heterocycles containing nitrogen;
4. Six-membered (cyclohexane) ring);
5. Benzene (aromatic six-membered) ring;
6. Fused pair of six-membered rings;
7. Bridged bicycle rings.

Several separate analyses were performed in this study. Thus, a Kohonen map was developed based on 57 of the most important proteins to classify them to certain classes.

In addition, the analysis of binding activity of each class of FDs and inside classes was done. The overall characteristics demonstrated that the most active FDs have the longest chain of substituents. Benzene, pyridine, and others aromatic rings also contributed to the highest binding activity, as well as the presence of cycle groups.

The lowest value of binding activity corresponds to pristine fullerene **FD168** (C60). Thus, the fullerene C60 possesses the lowest values of total surface area, molecular weight, rotatable bonds, electronegative atoms, sp3 atoms, polarizability, and topological diameter.

Then the CPANN analysis was done based on 27 descriptors, followed by the consensus model based on 10 descriptors. These models highlighted the importance of the following descriptors. It was shown that polarizability ($QPpolrz$), topological diameter (TD), total surface area, non H-atoms, and mol. weight are highly correlated with binding activity. These descriptors were used for characterization of pharmacokinetic events. The number of rotatable bonds descriptor contains information on a compound's conformational space and is highly correlated with binding activity of FDs. This descriptor characterizes the pharmacodynamic events dependent on interaction with biological targets.

In the study the analysis of 25 drug-like descriptors was made and it was shown how descriptors related to sp3 atoms and stereo centers, inversely correlated with aromatic atoms, helped to separate the hydrogenated (saturated) FDs from unsaturated. This information might be useful for selection of FDs for hydrogen storage technology when at the stage of searching for proper FDs. In addition, the role of LogP was analyzed and how it influences on the binding activity of FDs.

The results obtained in this study paves the way to study the clusters of proteins responsible for different diseases. Moreover, the investigation of clusters of different proteins enable the prediction of potential FDs as antiviral agents, enzyme inhibitors, ion channel blockers, neuroprotective agents, DNA breakers, photosensitizers in photodynamic therapy, fullerene-specific antibodies and nucleic acid binders, and free radical scavengers. The heatmap of 169 FDs related to 1117 proteins enables the exploration of the possible side effects of FDs in living organisms.

Supplementary Materials: The following are available online at http://www.mdpi.com/2079-4991/10/1/90/s1. Table S1. The list of 169 FDs with SMILE codes, molecular formula, indication of saturation (S), and binding activity (Av_Bscores values). S2–S61; Tables S2–S8. The classification of FDs dependent on type of bond of substituent groups attached to the fullerene C60 core. S62–S87; Table S2. GROUP 1: FDs with functional groups attached to the C60 core with single bond, with indication of the level of binding activity. S62–S63; Table S3. GROUP 2: FDs with functional groups attached to the C60 core with cyclopropane three-membered ring, with indication of the level of binding activity. S64–S69; Table S4. GROUP 3: FDs contained the substituent groups attached to the C60 core with pyrrolidine (five-membered ring) or pyridine (six-membered) heterocycles containing nitrogen, with indication of the level of binding activity. S70–S74; Table S5. GROUP 4: FDs contained the substituent groups attached to the C60 core with six-membered (cyclohexane) ring) with indication of the level of binding activity. S75–S77; Table S6. GROUP 5: FDs contained the substituent groups attached to the C60 core with benzene (aromatic six-membered) ring, with indication of the level of binding activity. S78–S85; Table S7. GROUP 6: FDs contained the FDs substituent s attached to the C60 core with fused pair of six-membered rings, with indication of the level of binding activity. S86; Table S8. GROUP 7: FDs contained the FDs substituent groups attached to the C60 core with bridged bicycle rings, with indication of the level of binding activity. S87; Table S9. Correlation between 27 descriptors (25 drug-like descriptors plus ($QPpolrz$ + TD)) and Bscores with correlation coefficients greater than 0.6. S113; Table S10. The differences between saturated and non-saturated fullerene derivatives. S114–S116; Figure 1S. The differences in binding activity (ΔBscores) between the most active FDs and pristine fullerene C_{60}. S88; Figure 2S. The architecture of CPANN. S90; (1). The list of considered proteins. S89; (2). The detailed description of neural networks used in the study. S90–S91; (3). Selection of the most significant proteins. S92.

Author Contributions: Data curation, B.R.; Formal analysis, K.V.; Supervision, M.N.; Writing—original draft, N.F. All authors have read and agreed to the published version of the manuscript.

Funding: This research received no external funding

Acknowledgments: Authors thank the Slovenian Ministry of Higher Education, Science and Technology (ARRS grant P1-017). This work is supported in part by the National Science Foundation under CHE-1800476 Award, ND EPSCoR Award #IIA-1355466 and by the State of North Dakota.

Conflicts of Interest: The authors declare no conflicts of interest.

References

1. Lalwani, G.; Sitharaman, B.J. Multifunctional fullerene and metallofullerene based nanobiomaterials. *Nano LIFE* **2013**, *3*. [CrossRef]
2. Xiao, L.; Takada, H.; Gan, X.H.; Miwa, N. The water-soluble fullerene derivative "Radical Sponge" exerts cytoprotective action against UVA irradiation but not visible-light-catalyzed cytotoxicity in human skin keratinocytes. *Bioorg. Med. Chem. Lett.* **2006**, *16*, 1590–1595. [CrossRef] [PubMed]
3. Djordjevic, A.; Srdjenovic, B.; Seke, M.; Petrovic, D.; Injac, R.; Mrdjanovic, J. Review of Synthesis and Antioxidant Potential of Fullerenol Nanoparticles. *J. Nanomater.* **2015**, *15*. [CrossRef]
4. Li, J.; Guan, M.; Wang, T.; Zhen, M.; Zhao, F.; Shu, C.; Wang, C. Gd@C_{82}-(ethylenediamine)$_8$ Nanoparticle: A New High-Efficiency Water-Soluble ROS Scavenger. *ACS Appl. Mater. Interfaces* **2016**, *8*, 25770–25776. [CrossRef] [PubMed]
5. Jacevic, V.; Djordjevic, A.; Srdjenovic, B.; Milic-Tores, V.; Segrt, Z.; Dragojevic-Simic, V.; Kuca, K. Fullerenol nanoparticles prevents doxorubicin-induced acute hepatotoxicity in rats. *Exp. Mol. Pathol.* **2017**, *102*, 360–369. [CrossRef] [PubMed]
6. Castro, E.; Hernandez Garcia, A.; Zavala, G.; Echegoyen, L. Fullerenes in biology and medicine. *J. Mater. Chem. B* **2017**, *5*, 6523–6535. [CrossRef] [PubMed]
7. Tzirakis, D.M.; Orfanopoulos, M. Radical Reactions of Fullerenes: From Synthetic Organic Chemistry to Materials Science and Biology. *Chem. Rev.* **2013**, *113*, 5262–5321. [CrossRef]
8. Mashino, T.; Okuda, K.; Hirota, T.; Hirobe, M.; Nagano, T.; Mochizuki, M. Inhibition of E. coli growth by fullerene derivatives and inhibition mechanism. *Bioorg. Med. Chem. Lett.* **1999**, *9*, 2959–2962. [CrossRef]
9. Friedman, S.H.; DeCamp, D.L.; Sijbesma, R.P.; Srdanov, G.; Wudl, F.; Kenyon, G.L. Inhibition of the HIV-1 protease by fullerene derivatives: Model building studies and experimental verification. *J. Am. Chem. Soc.* **1993**, *115*, 6506–6509. [CrossRef]
10. Ray, A. Fullerene (C60) Molecule—A Review. *Asian J. Pharm. Res.* **2012**, *2*, 48.
11. Bakry, R.; Vallant, R.M.; Najam-ul-Haq, M.; Rainer, M.; Szabo, Z.; Huck, C.W.; Bonn, G.K. Medicinal applications of fullerenes. *Int. J. Nanomed.* **2007**, *2*, 639–649.
12. Marchesan, S.; Da Ros, T.; Spalluto, G.; Balzarinib, J.; Pratoa, M. Anti-HIV properties of cationic fullerene derivatives. *Bioorg. Med. Chem. Lett.* **2005**, *15*, 3615–3618. [CrossRef]
13. Mashino, T.; Shimotohno, K.; Ikegami, N.; Nishikawa, D.; Okuda, K.; Takahashi, K.; Nakamura, S.; Mochizuki, M. Human immunodeficiency virus-reverse transcriptase inhibition and hepatitis C virus RNA-dependent RNA polymerase inhibition activities of fullerene derivatives. *Bioorg. Med. Chem. Lett.* **2005**, *15*, 1107–1109. [CrossRef] [PubMed]
14. Mengdan, Q.; Yaming, S.; Shanshan, G.; Hao, Z.; Song, W. Structural Basis of Fullerene Derivatives as Novel Potent Inhibitors of Protein Tyrosine Phosphatase 1B: Insight into the Inhibitory Mechanism through Molecular Modeling Studies. *J. Chem. Inf. Model.* **2016**, *56*, 2024–2034. [CrossRef]
15. Kang, S.; Mauter, M.S.; Elimelech, M.C. Microbial cycotoxicity of carbon-based nanomaterials: Implications for the river water and waste water effluent. *Environ. Sci. Technol.* **2009**, *43*, 2648–2653. [CrossRef] [PubMed]
16. Lyon, D.Y.; Adams, L.K.; Faulkner, J.C.; Alvarez, J.J. Antibacterial activity of fullerene water suspension: Effects of preparation methods and particle size. *Environ. Sci. Technol.* **2006**, *40*, 4360–4366. [CrossRef] [PubMed]

17. Fortner, J.D.; Lyon, D.Y.; Sayes, C.M.; Boyd, A.M.; Falkner, J.C.; Horze, E.M.; Hughes, J.B. C60 in water: Nano crystal formation and microbial response. *Environ. Sci. Technol.* **2005**, *39*, 4307–4316. [CrossRef]
18. Das, R.; Vecitis, C.D.; Schulze, A.; Cao, B.; Ismail, A.F.; Lu, X.; Ramakrishna, S. Recent advances in nanomaterials for water protection and monitoring. *Chem. Soc. Rev.* **2017**, *46*, 6946–7020. [CrossRef]
19. Arbogast, J.W.; Foote, C.S.; Kao, M. Electron transfer to triplet fullerene C60. *J. Am. Chem. Soc.* **1992**, *114*, 2277–2279. [CrossRef]
20. Nimibofa, A.; Ebelegi, A.; Abasi, C.; Donbebe, W. Fullerenes: Synthesis and Applications. *J. Mater. Sci.* **2018**, *7*, 22–33. [CrossRef]
21. Gokhale, M.; Somani, R. Fullerenes: Chemistry and Its Applications. *Mini-Rev. Org. Chem.* **2015**, *12*, 355–366. [CrossRef]
22. Aschberger, K.; Johnston, H.J.; Stone, V.; Aitken, R.J.; Tran, C.L.; Hankin, S.M.; Peters, S.A.; Christensen, F.M. Review of fullerene toxicity and exposure–appraisal of a human health risk assessment, based on open literature. *Regul. Toxicol. Pharmacol.* **2010**, *58*, 455–473. [CrossRef] [PubMed]
23. Bhabra, G.; Sood, A.; Fisher, B.; Cartwright, L.; Saunders, M.; Evans, W.H.; Surprenant, A.; Lopez-Castejon, G.; Mann, S.; Davis, S.A.; et al. Nanoparticles can cause DNA damage across a cellular barrier. *Nat. Nanotechnol.* **2009**, *4*, 876–883. [CrossRef]
24. Gong, M.; Yang, H.; Zhang, S.; Yang, Y.; Zhang, D.; Qi, Y.; Zou, L. Superparamagnetic core/shell GoldMag nanoparticles: Size-, concentration- and time-dependent cellular nanotoxicity on human umbilical vein endothelial cells and the suitable conditions for magnetic resonance imaging. *J. Nanobiotechnol.* **2015**, *13*, 1–16. [CrossRef] [PubMed]
25. Puzyn, T.; Gajewicz, A.; Leszczynska, D.; Leszczynski, J. Nanomaterials—the Next Great Challenge for QSAR Modelers. In *Recent Advances in QSAR Studies: Methods and Applications*; Puzyn, T., Leszczynski, J., Cronin, M.T., Eds.; Springer: London, UK; New York, NY, USA, 2010; Chapter 14; pp. 383–410.
26. Puzyn, T.; Leszczynska, D.; Leszczynski, J. Toward the Development of "Nano-QSARs": Advances and Challenges. *Small* **2009**, *5*, 2494–2509. [CrossRef]
27. Toropov, A.A.; Benfenati, E. SMILES in QSPR/QSAR Modeling: Results and Perspectives. *Curr. Drug Discov. Technol.* **2007**, *4*, 77–116. [CrossRef]
28. Bonnefoi, M.S.; Belanger, S.E.; Devlin, D.J.; Doerrer, N.G.; Embry, M.R.; Fukushima, S.; Harpur, E.S.; Hines, R.N.; Holsapple, M.P.; Kim, J.H.; et al. Human and Environmental Health Challenges for the Next Decade (2010–2020). *Crit. Rev. Toxicol.* **2010**, *40*, 893–911. [CrossRef]
29. Moore, M.N. Do Nanoparticles Present Ecotoxicological Risks for the Health of the Aquatic Environment? *Environ. Int.* **2006**, *32*, 967–976. [CrossRef]
30. Tsuji, J.S.; Maynard, A.D.; Howard, P.C.; James, J.T.; Lam, C.W.; Warheit, D.B.; Santamaria, A.B. Research Strategies for Safety Evaluation of Nanomaterials, Part IV: Risk Assessment of Nanoparticles. *Toxicol. Sci.* **2006**, *89*, 42–50. [CrossRef]
31. Worth, A. The role of QSAR methodology in the regulatory assessment of chemicals. In *Recent Advances in QSAR Studies: Methods and Applications*; Puzyn, T., Leszczynski, J., Cronin, M.T., Eds.; Springer: London, UK; New York, NY, USA, 2010; Chapter 13; pp. 367–382. [CrossRef]
32. Rivera Gil, P.; Oberdörster, G.; Elder, A.; Puntes, V.; Parak, W. Correlating physico-chemical with toxicological properties of nanoparticles: The present and the future. *ACS Nano* **2010**, *4*, 5527–5531. [CrossRef]
33. Durdagi, S.; Mavromoustakos, T.; Papadopulos, M. 3D QSAR CoMFA/CoMSIA, molecular docking and molecular dynamics studies of fullerene-based HIV-1 PR inhibitors. *Bioorg. Med. Chem. Lett.* **2008**, *18*, 6283–6289. [CrossRef] [PubMed]
34. Durdagi, S.; Mavromoustakos, T.; Chronakis, N.; Papadopoulos, M. Computational design of novel fullerene analogs as potential HIV 1 PR inhibitors: Analysis of the binding interactions between fullerene Inhibitors and HIV 1 PR residues using 3D QSAR, molecular docking and molecular dynamics simulations. *Bioorg. Med. Chem. Lett.* **2008**, *16*, 9957–9974. [CrossRef] [PubMed]
35. Martin, D.; Karelson, M. The quantitative structure activity relationships for predicting HIV protease inhibition by substituted fullerenes. *Lett. Drug. Des. Discov.* **2010**, *7*, 587–595. [CrossRef]
36. Shultz, M.D. Two Decades under the Influence of the Rule of Five and the Changing Properties of Approved Oral Drugs. *J. Med. Chem.* **2018**, *62*, 1701–1714. [CrossRef]
37. Ursu, O.; Rayan, A.; Goldblum, A.; Oprea, T.I. Understanding drug-likeness. *WIREs Comput. Mol. Sci.* **2011**, *1*, 760–781. [CrossRef]

38. Oprea, T.I. Property distribution of drug-related chemical databases. *J. Comput. Aided Mol. Des.* **2000**, *14*, 251–264. [CrossRef]
39. Worth, A. The future of *in silico* chemical safety ... and beyond. *Computat. Toxicol.* **2019**, *10*, 60–62. [CrossRef]
40. Ahmed, L.; Rasulev, B.; Kar, S.; Krupa, P.; Mozolewska, M.A.; Leszczynski, J. Inhibitors or toxins? Large Library Target-specific Screening of Fullerene-based Nanoparticles for Drug Design Purpose. *Nanoscale* **2017**, *9*, 10263–10276. [CrossRef]
41. Burley, S.; Berman, H.; Bhikadiya, C.; Bi, C.; Chen, L.; Di Costanzo, L.; Christie, C.; Dalenberg, K.; Duarte, J.M.; Dutta, S.; et al. RCSB Protein Data Bank: Biological macromolecular structures enabling research and education in fundamental biology, biomedicine, biotechnology and energy. *Nucleic Acids Res.* **2019**, *47*, D464–D474. [CrossRef]
42. Sander, T.; Freyss, J.; Korff, M.; Rufener, C. DataWarrior: An Open-Source Program for Chemistry Aware Data Visualization and Analysis. *J. Chem. Inf. Model.* **2015**, *55*, 460–473. [CrossRef]
43. Zupan, J.; Novič, M.; Ruisainchez, I. Kohonen and Counterpropagation Artificial Neural Networks in Analytical Chemistry. *Chemometr. Intell. Lab. Syst.* **1997**, *38*, 1–23. [CrossRef]
44. Zupan, J.; Gasteiger, J. *Neural Networks in Chemistry and Drug Design*, 2nd ed.; Wiley-VCH Verlag GmbH: Weinheim, Germany, 1999.
45. Vračko, M.; Novič, M.; Zupan, J. Study of Structure-Toxicity Relationship by a Counter-propagation Neural Network. *Anal. Chim. Acta* **1999**, *384*, 319–332. [CrossRef]
46. Kohonen, T. *Self-Organizing Maps*; Springer: Berlin, Germany, 2001. [CrossRef]
47. Grošelj, N.; Van der Veer, G.; Tušar, M.; Vračko, M.; Novič, M. Verification of the Geological Origin of Bottled Mineral Water Using Artificial Neural Networks. *Food Chem.* **2010**, *118*, 941–947. [CrossRef]
48. Fowler, P.; Ceulemans, A. Electron deficiency of the fullerenes. *J. Phys. Chem.* **1995**, *99*, 508–510. [CrossRef]
49. Zeynalov, E.B.; Allen, N.S.; Salmanova, N.I. Radical scavenging efficiency of different fullerenes C60–C70 and fullerene soot. *Polym. Degrad. Stab.* **2009**, *94*, 1183–1189. [CrossRef]
50. Keller, T.; Pichota, A.; Yin, Z. A practical view of 'druggability'. *Curr. Opin. Chem. Biol.* **2006**, *10*, 357–361. [CrossRef]
51. Lipinski, C. Drug-like properties and the causes of poor solubility and poor permeability. *J. Pharmacol. Toxicol. Methods* **2000**, *44*, 3–25. [CrossRef]
52. Vistoli, G.; Pedretti, A.; Testa, B. Assessing Drug-likeness–What are we Missing? *Drug Discov. Today* **2008**, *13*, 285–294. [CrossRef]
53. Tropsha, A.; Gramatica, P.; Gombar Vijay, K. The Importance of Being Earnest: Validation is the Absolute Essential for Successful Application and Interpretation of QSPR Models. *Mol. Inform.* **2003**, *22*, 69–77. [CrossRef]
54. Gramatica, P. Principles of QSAR models validation: Internal and external. *Mol. Inform.* **2007**, *26*, 694–701. [CrossRef]
55. Mazzatorta, P.; Vračko, M.; Jezierska, A.; Benfenati, E. Modeling Toxicity by Using Supervised Kohonen Neural Networks. *J. Chem. Inf. Comput. Sci.* **2003**, *43*, 485–492. [CrossRef] [PubMed]
56. Ritchie, T.J.; Macdonald, S.J. The impact of aromatic ring count on compound developability–are too many aromatic rings a liability in drug design? *Drug Discov. Today* **2009**, *14*, 1011–1020. [CrossRef] [PubMed]
57. Matsson, P.; Doak, B.C.; Over, B.; Kihlberg, J. Cell Permeability beyond the Rule of 5. *Adv. Drug Deliv. Rev.* **2016**, *101*, 42–61. [CrossRef] [PubMed]
58. Godly, E.W.; Taylor, R. Nomenclature and Terminology of Fullerenes: A Preliminary Survey. *Pure Appl. Chem.* **1997**, *69*, 1411–1434. [CrossRef]
59. Powell, W.H.; Cozzi, F.; Moss, G.P.; Thilgen, C.; Hwu, R.J.-R.; Yerin, A. Nomenclature for the C60-*Ih* and C70-D5h(6) Fullerenes (IUPAC Recommendations 2002). *Pure Appl. Chem.* **2002**, *74*, 629–695. [CrossRef]
60. Lovering, F.; Bikker, J.; Humblet, C. Escape from Flatland: Increasing Saturation as an Approach to Improving Clinical Success. *J. Med. Chem.* **2009**, *52*, 6752–6756. [CrossRef]
61. Buseck, P.; Tsipursky, S.; Hettich, R. Fullerenes from the Geological Environment. *Science* **1992**, *257*, 215–217. [CrossRef]
62. Shabbir, M.; Hong-Liang, X.; Rong-Lin, Z.; Zhong-Min, S.; Abdullah GAl-Sehemi Ahmad, I. Quantum chemical design of nonlinear optical materials by sp^2-hybridized carbon nanomaterials: Issues and opportunities. *J. Mater. Chem. C* **2013**, *1*, 5439–5449. [CrossRef]

63. Ritchie, T.J.; Macdonald, S.J.F. Physicochemical Descriptors of Aromatic Character and Their Use in Drug Discovery. *J. Med. Chem.* **2014**, *57*, 7206–7215. [CrossRef]
64. Jagiello, K.; Grzonkowska, M.; Swirog, M.; Ahmed, L.; Rasulev, B.; Avramopoulos, A.; Papadopoulos, M.G.; Leszczynski, J.; Puzyn, T. Advantages and limitations of classic and 3D QSAR approaches in nano-QSAR studies based on biological activity of fullerene derivatives. *J. Nanopart. Res.* **2016**, *18*, 256. [CrossRef]
65. Turabekova, M.A.; Rasulev, B.F.; Dzhakhangirov, F.N.; Salikhov, S.I. Aconitum and Delphinium alkaloids: "Drug-likeness" descriptors related to toxic mode of action. *Environ. Toxicol. Pharmacol.* **2008**, *25*, 310–320. [CrossRef] [PubMed]

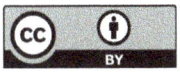

© 2020 by the authors. Licensee MDPI, Basel, Switzerland. This article is an open access article distributed under the terms and conditions of the Creative Commons Attribution (CC BY) license (http://creativecommons.org/licenses/by/4.0/).

MDPI
St. Alban-Anlage 66
4052 Basel
Switzerland
Tel. +41 61 683 77 34
Fax +41 61 302 89 18
www.mdpi.com

Nanomaterials Editorial Office
E-mail: nanomaterials@mdpi.com
www.mdpi.com/journal/nanomaterials

www.ingramcontent.com/pod-product-compliance
Lightning Source LLC
LaVergne TN
LVHW070608100526
838202LV00012B/592